Ben Stacy Jerrik (Ed.)

Segmentation Contractions

Ben Stacy Jerrik (Ed.)

Segmentation Contractions

Esophagus

Part Press

Imprint

Publisher:
Part Press is a trademark of
International Book Market Service Ltd., 17 Rue Meldrum, Beau Bassin, 1713-01 Mauritius
Email: info@bookmarketservice.com
Website: www.bookmarketservice.com

Published in 2011

Printed in: U.S.A., U.K., Germany. This book was not produced in Mauritius.

ISBN: 978-613-7-88792-9

Contents

Articles

References

Segmentation contractions

Segmentation contractions (or **movements**) are a type of gastric motility.

Unlike peristalsis, which predominates in the esophagus, **segmentation contractions** occur in the large intestine and small intestine, while predominating in the latter. While peristalsis involves one-way motion in the caudal direction, segmentation contractions move chyme in both directions, which allows greater mixing with the secretions of the intestines.

External links

- Physiology at MCG *6/6ch3/s6ch3_8* [1]
- Animation at colostate.edu [2]
- "Segmentation contraction [3]" at *Dorland's Medical Dictionary*

References

[1] http://www.lib.mcg.edu/edu/eshuphysio/program/section6/6ch3/s6ch3_8.htm
[2] http://www.vivo.colostate.edu/hbooks/pathphys/digestion/basics/gi_motility.html
[3] http://web.archive.org/web/20090616022448/http://www.mercksource.com/pp/us/cns/cns_hl_dorlands_split.jsp?pg=/ppdocs/us/common/dorlands/dorland/two/000023965.htm

Esophagus

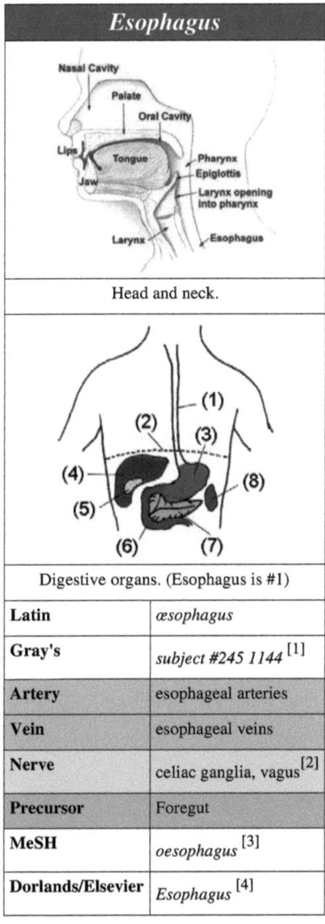

Head and neck.

Digestive organs. (Esophagus is #1)

Latin	*œsophagus*
Gray's	*subject #245 1144* [1]
Artery	esophageal arteries
Vein	esophageal veins
Nerve	celiac ganglia, vagus[2]
Precursor	Foregut
MeSH	*oesophagus* [3]
Dorlands/Elsevier	*Esophagus* [4]

The **esophagus** (or **oesophagus**) is an organ in vertebrates which consists of a muscular tube through which food passes from the pharynx to the stomach. During swallowing, food passes from the mouth through the pharynx into the esophagus and travels via peristalsis to the stomach. The word *esophagus* is derived from the Latin *œsophagus*, which derives from the Greek word *oisophagos* , lit. "entrance for eating." In humans the esophagus is continuous with the laryngeal part of the pharynx at the level of the C6 vertebra. The esophagus passes through posterior mediastinum in thorax and enters abdomen through a hole in the diaphragm at the level of the tenth thoracic vertebrae (T10). It is usually about 25–30 cm long depending on individual height. It is divided into cervical, thoracic and abdominal parts. Due to the inferior pharyngeal constrictor muscle, the entry to the esophagus opens only when swallowing or vomiting.

Histology

The layers of the esophagus are as follows:[5]

- *mucosa*
  - nonkeratinized *stratified squamous epithelium*: is rapidly turned over, and serves a protective effect due to the high volume transit of food, saliva and mucus.
  - *lamina propria*: sparse.
  - *muscularis mucosae*: smooth muscle
- *submucosa*: Contains the mucous secreting glands (esophageal glands), and connective structures termed papillae.
- *muscularis externa* (or "muscularis propria"): composition varies in different parts of the esophagus, to correspond with the conscious control over swallowing in the upper portions and the autonomic control in the lower portions:
  - *upper third, or superior part*: striated muscle
  - *middle third, smooth muscle and striated muscle*
  - *inferior third*: predominantly smooth muscle
- *adventitia*

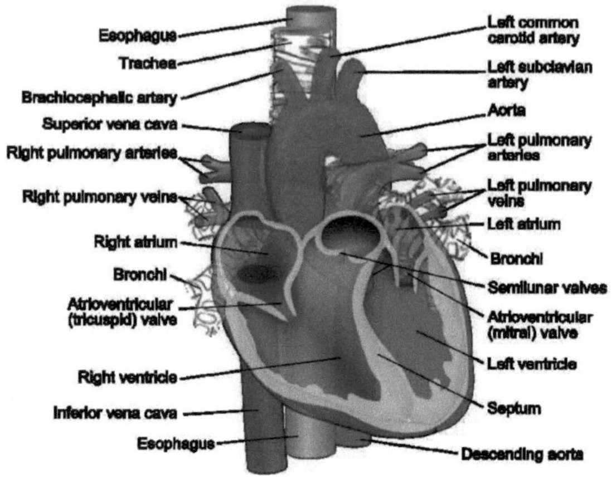

Course of the esophagus (anterior view), showing it passing posteriorly to the trachea and the heart.

Esophageal constrictions

Normally, the esophagus has three anatomic constrictions at the following levels;[6] [7]

- At the esophageal inlet, where the pharynx joins the esophagus, behind the cricoid cartilage (14-16 cm from the incisor teeth).
- Where its anterior surface is crossed by the aortic arch and the left bronchus (25-27 cm from the incisor teeth).
- Where it pierces the diaphragm (36-38 cm from the incisor teeth).

The distances from the incisor teeth are important as is useful for diagnostic endoscopic procedures.

Gastroesophageal junction

The junction between the oesophagus and the stomach (the **gastroesophageal junction** or **GE junction**) is not actually considered a valve, although it is sometimes called the cardiac sphincter, cardia or cardias, it actually better resembles a structure.

In much of the gastrointestinal tract, smooth muscles contract in sequence to produce a peristaltic wave which forces a ball of food (called a bolus) while in the esophagus. In humans, peristalsis is found in the contraction of smooth muscles to propel contents through the digestive tract.

In other animals

In most fish, the oesophagus is extremely short, primarily due to the length of the pharynx (which is associated with the gills). However, some fish, including lampreys, chimaeras, and lungfish, have no true stomach, so that the esophagus effectively runs from the pharynx directly to the intestine, and is therefore somewhat longer.[8]

In tetrapods, the pharynx is much shorter, and the esophagus correspondingly longer, than in fish. In amphibians, sharks and rays, the esophageal epithelium is ciliated, helping to wash food along, in addition to the action of muscular peristalsis. In the majority of vertebrates, the esophagus is simply a connecting tube, but in birds, it is extended towards the lower end to form a crop for storing food before it enters the true stomach.[8]

A structure with the same name is often found in invertebrates, including molluscs and arthropods, connecting the oral cavity with the stomach.

See also

- Esophageal disease
- Esophageal sphincter

Additional images

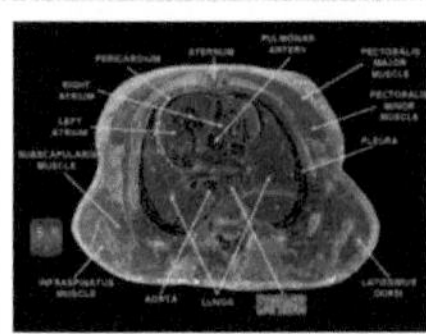

Esophagus

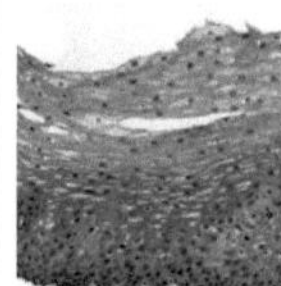

H&E stain of biopsy of normal esophagus showing the stratified squamous cell epithelium

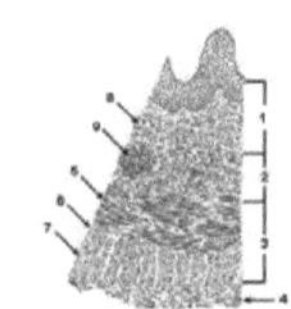

Layers of the esophagus.

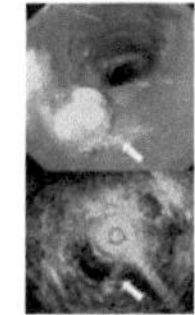

Mid-esophageal mass

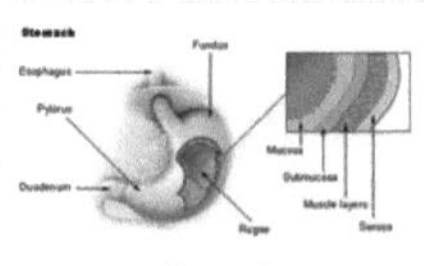

Stomach

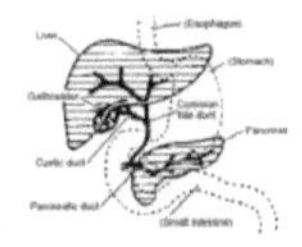

Accessory digestive system.

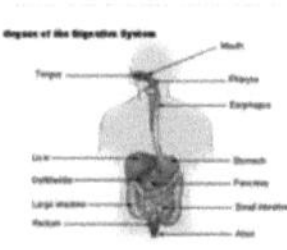

Organs of the digestive tract.

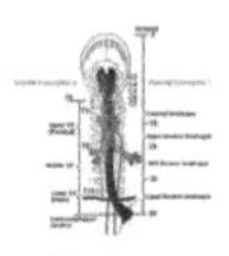

Esophagus

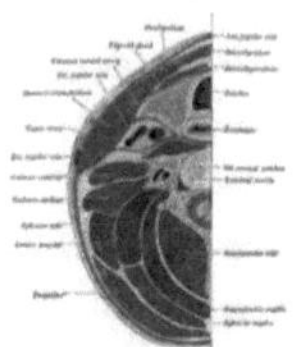

Section of the neck at about the level of the sixth cervical vertebra.

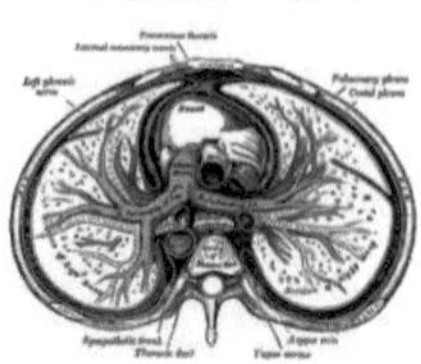

Transverse section of thorax, showing relations of pulmonary artery.

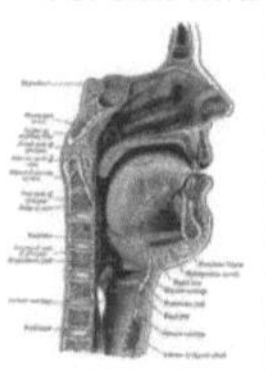

Sagittal section of nose mouth, pharynx, and larynx.

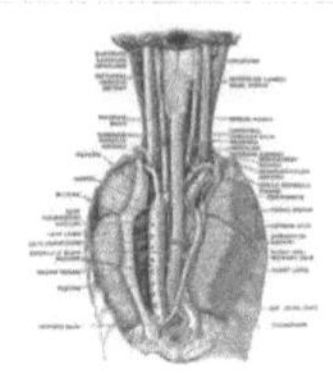

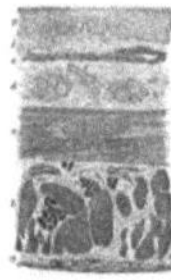

Section of the human esophagus. Moderately magnified.

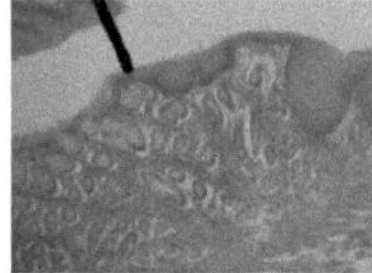

Microscopic shot of a cross section of human gastroesophageal junction wall.

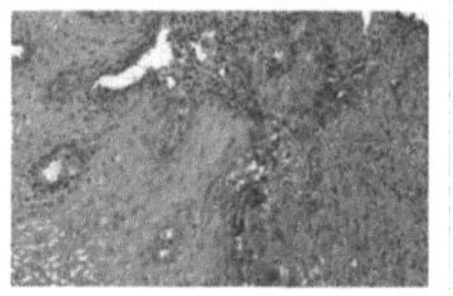

Micrograph of herpes esophagitis. H&E stain.

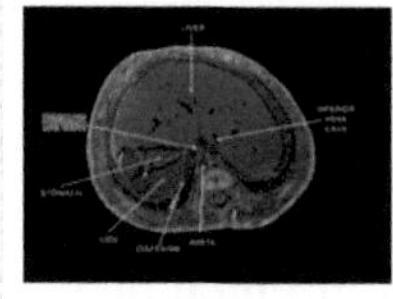

Esophagus

References

[1] http://education.yahoo.com/reference/gray/subjects/subject?id=245#p1144

[2] Physiology at MCG *6/6ch2/s6ch2_30* (http://www.lib.mcg.edu/edu/eshuphysio/program/section6/6ch2/s6ch2_30.htm)

[3] http://www.nlm.nih.gov/cgi/mesh/2011/MB_cgi?mode=&term=oesophagus

[4] http://www.mercksource.com/pp/us/cns/cns_hl_dorlands_split.jsp?pg=/ppdocs/us/common/dorlands/dorland/three/000036999.htm

[5] Histology at BU *10801loa* (http://www.bu.edu/histology/p/10801loa.htm)

[6] Snell, Richard (2007). *Clinical anatomy by regions* (http://books.google.com/books?id=7SZWRe2OBlgC&pg=PA129). Lippincott Williams & Wilkins. p. 129. ISBN 9780781764049. .

[7] Schünke, Michael; Schulte, Erik; Schumacher, Udo; Ross, Lawrence; Lamperti, Edward (2006). *Atlas of anatomy: neck and internal organs* (http://books.google.com/books?id=n0jqG0Lv2CAC&pg=PA70). Thieme. p. 70. ISBN 9781588904430. .

[8] Romer, Alfred Sherwood; Parsons, Thomas S. (1977). *The Vertebrate Body*. Philadelphia, PA: Holt-Saunders International. pp. 344–345. ISBN 0-03-910284-X.

External links

- Virtual Slidebox at Univ. Iowa *Slide 449* (http://www.path.uiowa.edu/cgi-bin-pub/vs/fpx_gen.cgi?slide=449&viewer=java&view=0&lay=nlm)
- Esophagus Foreign Body (http://rad.usuhs.edu/medpix/kiosk_image.html?mode=cow_viewer&pt_id=14011&imageid=56622#pic) MedPix Radiology Teaching File

bjn:Rakungan

Peristalsis

Peristalsis is a radially symmetrical contraction and relaxation of muscles which propagates in a wave down the muscular tube, in an anterograde fashion. In humans, peristalsis is found in the contraction of smooth muscles to propel contents through the digestive tract. Earthworms use a similar mechanism to drive their locomotion. The word is derived from New Latin and comes from the Greek *peristallein*, "to wrap around," from *peri-*, "around" + *stallein*, "to place".

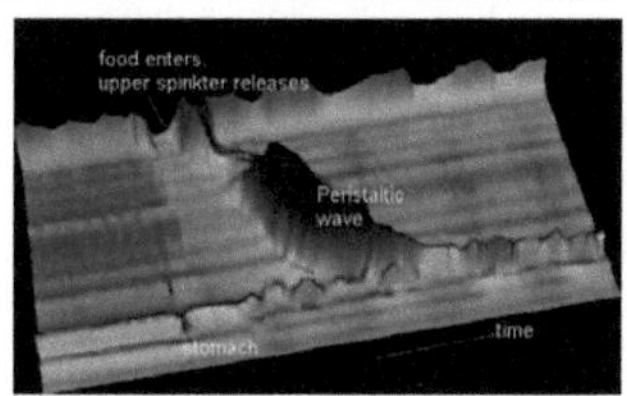

A time-space diagram of a peristaltic wave after a water swallow. High pressure values are red, zero pressure is blue-green. The ridge in the upper part of the picture is the high pressure of the upper esophageal sphincter which only opens for a short time to let water pass.

In much of the gastrointestinal tract, smooth muscles contract in sequence to produce a peristaltic wave which forces a ball of food (called a bolus while in the esophagus and gastrointestinal tract and chyme in the stomach) along the gastrointestinal tract. Peristaltic movement is initiated by circular smooth muscles contracting behind the chewed material to prevent it from moving back into the mouth, followed by a contraction of longitudinal smooth muscles which pushes the digested food forward. Catastalsis is a related intestinal muscle process.[1]

Esophagus

After food is chewed into a bolus, it is swallowed and moved through the esophagus. Smooth muscles contract behind the bolus to prevent it from being squeezed back into the mouth. Then rhythmic, unidirectional waves of contractions will work to rapidly force the food into the stomach. This process works in one direction only and its sole purpose is to move food from the mouth into the stomach.[2]

In the esophagus, two types of peristalsis occur.

- First, there is a **primary peristaltic wave** which occurs when the bolus enters the esophagus during swallowing. The primary peristaltic wave forces the bolus down the esophagus and into the stomach in a wave lasting about 8–9 seconds. The wave travels down to the stomach even if the bolus of food descends at a greater rate than the wave itself, and will continue even if for some reason the bolus gets stuck further up the esophagus.
- In the event that the bolus gets stuck or moves slower than the primary peristaltic wave (as can happen when it is poorly lubricated), stretch receptors in the esophageal lining are stimulated and a local reflex response causes a **secondary peristaltic wave** around the bolus, forcing it further down the esophagus, and these secondary waves will continue indefinitely until the bolus enters the stomach.

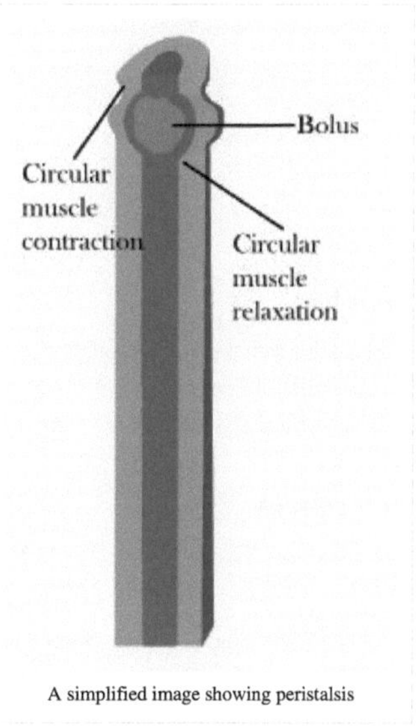

A simplified image showing peristalsis

Esophageal peristalsis is typically assessed by performing an esophageal motility study.

Small intestine

Once processed and digested by the stomach, the milky chyme is squeezed through the pyloric sphincter into the small intestine. Once past the stomach a typical peristaltic wave will only last for a few seconds, travelling at only a few centimeters per second. Its primary purpose is to mix the chyme in the intestine rather than to move it forward in the intestine. Through this process of mixing and continued digestion and absorption of nutrients, the chyme gradually works its way through the small intestine to the large intestine. [3]

During vomiting the propulsion of food up the esophagus and out the mouth comes from contraction of the abdominal muscles; peristalsis does not reverse in the esophagus.

As opposed to the more continuous peristalsis of the small intestines, faecal contents are propelled into the large intestine by periodic mass movements. These mass movements occur one to three times per day in the large intestines and colon, and help propel the contents from the large intestine through the colon to the rectum.

Earthworms

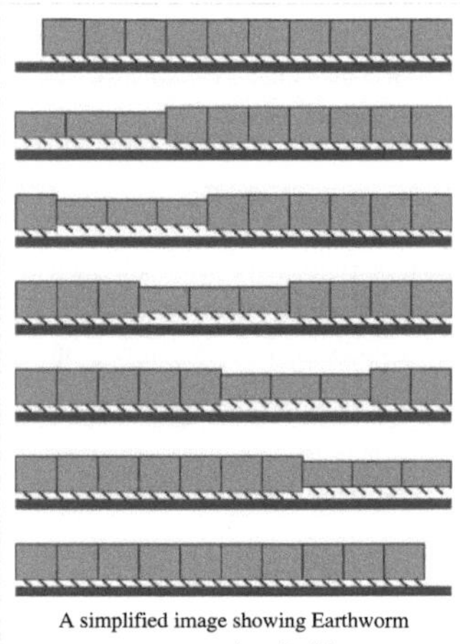

A simplified image showing Earthworm movement via peristalsis

The earthworm is a limbless annelid worm with a hydrostatic skeleton that moves by means of peristalsis. This hydrostatic skeleton consists of an extensible body wall surrounded by a fluid-filled body cavity. The worm moves by radially constricting the anterior portion of its body, resulting in an increase in length via hydrostatic pressure. This constricted region propagates posteriorly along the worm's body. As a result, each segment is extended forward, then relaxes and re-contacts the substrate, with hair-like setae preventing backwards slipping.[4] Earthworms increase four orders of magnitude during their lifetime and during this period the dimensions increase according to geometric similarity, or 'isometry'. Unlike rigid skeletons which cannot exhibit both geometric and stress similarity, the hydrostatic skeleton can maintain both forms which may be due to decoupling of weight and skeletal function.[4]

See also

- Peristaltic pump - Mechanical device that uses peristaltic action to drive fluids
- Catastalsis - Downward wave of contraction occurring in the gastrointestinal tract during digestion
- Basal electrical rhythm - Slow wave of electrical activity that can initiate contraction

References

[1] Marieb, Elaine N. & Hoehn, Katja "Human Anatomy & Physiology" 8th Ed., Benjamin Cummings/Pearson, 2010
[2] Marieb, Elaine N. & Hoehn, Katja "Human Anatomy & Physiology" 8th Ed., Benjamin Cummings/Pearson, 2010
[3] Marieb, Elaine N. & Hoehn, Katja "Human Anatomy & Physiology" 8th Ed., Benjamin Cummings/Pearson, 2010
[4] Quillin, K.J. Ontogenetic Scaling of Hydrostatic Skeletons: Geometric, Static, Stress and Dynamic Stress Scaling of the Earthworm Lubricus Terrestris

See also Peristaltic Linear Motion. A flexible tube constricted with rollers which produces linear motion when pressurised with air or liquids.

External links

- Interactive 3D display of swallow waves at menne-biomed.de (http://www.menne-biomed.de/swallow/jswallow3d.php)
- MeSH *Peristalsis* (http://www.nlm.nih.gov/cgi/mesh/2011/MB_cgi?mode=&term=Peristalsis)
- Physiology at MCG *6/6ch3/s6ch3_9* (http://www.lib.mcg.edu/edu/eshuphysio/program/section6/6ch3/s6ch3_9.htm)
- Overview at colostate.edu (http://www.vivo.colostate.edu/hbooks/pathphys/digestion/basics/peristalsis.html)

Small intestine

Small Intestine	
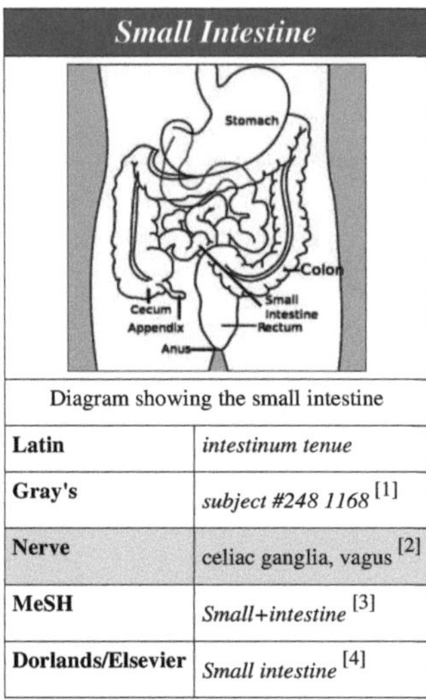	
Diagram showing the small intestine	
Latin	*intestinum tenue*
Gray's	*subject #248 1168* [1]
Nerve	celiac ganglia, vagus [2]
MeSH	*Small+intestine* [3]
Dorlands/Elsevier	*Small intestine* [4]

The **small intestine** is the part of the gastrointestinal tract following the stomach and followed by the large intestine, and is where much of the digestion and absorption of food takes place. In invertebrates such as worms, the terms "gastrointestinal tract" and "large intestine" are often used to describe the entire intestine. This article is primarily about the human gut, though the information about its processes is directly applicable to most placental mammals. The primary function of the small intestine is the absorption of nutrients and minerals found in food. [5] (A major exception to this are cows; for information about digestion in cows and other similar mammals, see ruminants.)

Size and divisions

The average length of the small intestine in an adult human male is 22 feet 6 inches (6.9 m), and in the adult female 23 feet 4 inches (7.1 m). However, it can vary greatly, from as short as 15 feet (4.6 m) to as long as 32 feet (9.8m).[6] [7] It is approximately 2.5–3 cm in diameter.

The small intestine is divided into three structural parts:

- **Duodenum**
- **Jejunum**
- **Ileum**

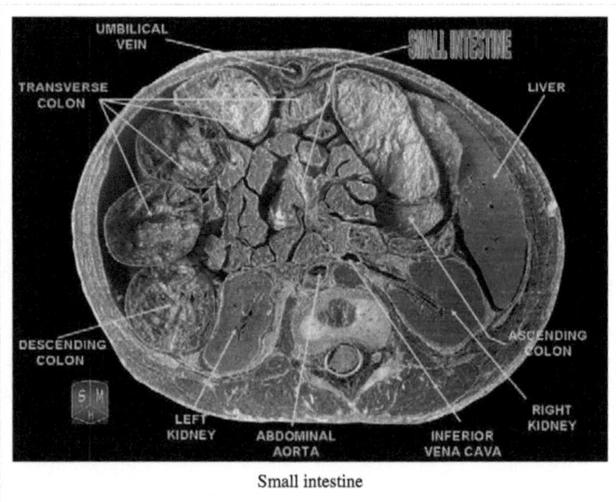

Small intestine

Histology

The three sections of the small intestine look similar to each other at a microscopic level, but there are some important differences. The parts of the intestine are as follows:

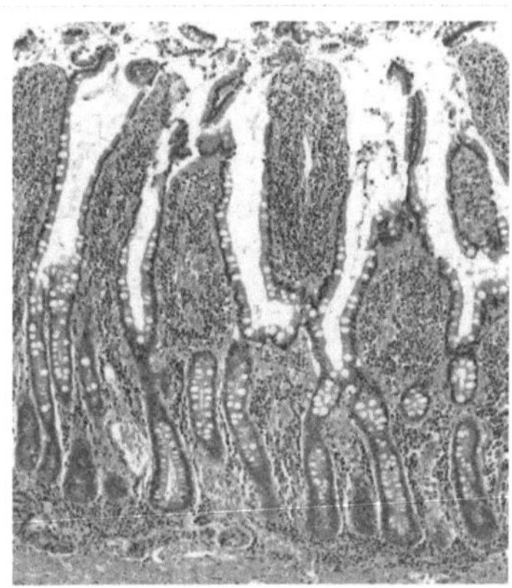

Micrograph of the **small intestine** mucosa showing the intestinal villi and crypts of Lieberkühn.

Layer	Duodenum	Jejunum	Ileum
serosa	normal	normal	normal
muscularis externa	longitudinal and circular layers, with Auerbach's (myenteric) plexus in between	same as duodenum	same as duodenum
submucosa	Brunner's glands and Meissner's (submucosal) plexus	no BG	no BG
mucosa: muscularis mucosae	normal	normal	normal
mucosa: lamina propria	no PP	no PP	Peyer's patches
mucosa: intestinal epithelium	simple columnar. Contains goblet cells, Paneth cells	Similar to duodenum. Villi very long.	Similar to duodenum. Villi very short.

Digestion and absorption

Food from the stomach is allowed into the duodenum by a muscle called the pylorus, or pyloricistalsis.

Digestion

The small intestine is where most chemical digestion takes place. Most of the digestive enzymes that act in the small intestine are secreted by the pancreas and enter the small intestine via the pancreatic duct. The enzymes enter the small intestine in response to the hormone cholecystokinin, which is produced in the small intestine in response to the presence of nutrients. The hormone secretin also causes bicarbonate to be released into the small intestine from the pancreas in order to neutralize the potentially harmful acid coming from the stomach.

The three major classes of nutrients that undergo digestion are proteins, lipids (fats) and carbohydrates:

- Proteins and peptides are degraded into amino acids. Chemical breakdown begins in the stomach and continues in the large intestine. Proteolytic enzymes, including trypsin and chymotrypsin, are secreted by the pancreas and cleave proteins into smaller peptides. Carboxypeptidase, which is a pancreatic brush border enzyme, splits one amino acid at a time. Aminopeptidase and dipeptidase free the end amino acid products.

- Lipids (fats) are degraded into fatty acids and glycerol. Pancreatic lipase breaks down triglycerides into free fatty acids and monoglycerides. Pancreatic lipase works with the help of the salts from the bile secreted by the liver and the gall bladder. Bile salts attach to triglycerides to help emulsify them, which aids access by pancreatic lipase. This occurs because the lipase is water-soluble but the fatty triglycerides are hydrophobic and tend to orient towards each other and away from the watery intestinal surroundings. The bile salts are the "main man" that holds the triglycerides in the watery surroundings until the lipase can break them into the smaller components that are able to enter the villi for absorption.
- Some carbohydrates are degraded into simple sugars, or monosaccharides (e.g., glucose). Pancreatic amylase breaks down some carbohydrates (notably starch) into oligosaccharides. Other carbohydrates pass undigested into the large intestine and further handling by intestinal bacteria. Brush border enzymes take over from there. The most important brush border enzymes are dextrinase and glucoamylase which further break down oligosaccharides. Other brush border enzymes are maltase, sucrase and lactase. Lactase is absent in most adult humans and for them lactose, like most poly-saccharides are not digested in the small intestine. Some carbohydrates, such as cellulose, are not digested at all, despite being made of multiple glucose units, this is because the cellulose is made out of beta-glucose, making the inter-monosaccharidal bindings different from the ones present in starch, which consists of alpha-glucose. Humans lack the enzyme for splitting the beta-glucose-bonds, something reserved for herbivores and bacteria from the large intestine.

Absorption

Digested food is now able to pass into the blood vessels in the wall of the intestine through the process of diffusion. The small intestine is the site where most of the nutrients from ingested food are absorbed. The inner wall, or mucosa, of the small intestine is lined with simple columnar epithelial tissue. Structurally, the mucosa is covered in wrinkles or folds called plicae circulares, which are considered permanent features in the wall of the organ. They are distinct from rugae which are considered non-permanent or temporary allowing for distention and contraction. From the plicae circulares project microscopic finger-like pieces of tissue called villi (Latin for "shaggy hair"). The individual epithelial cells also have finger-like projections known as microvilli. The function of the plicae circulares, the villi and the microvilli is to increase the amount of surface area available for the absorption of nutrients.

Each villus has a network of capillaries and fine lymphatic vessels called lacteals close to its surface. The epithelial cells of the villi transport nutrients from the lumen of the intestine into these capillaries (amino acids and carbohydrates) and lacteals (lipids). The absorbed substances are transported via the blood vessels to different organs of the body where they are used to build complex substances such as the proteins required by our body. The food that remains undigested and unabsorbed passes into the large intestine.

Absorption of the majority of nutrients takes place in the jejunum, with the following notable exceptions:

- Iron is absorbed in the duodenum.
- Vitamin B12 and bile salts are absorbed in the terminal ileum.
- Water and lipids are absorbed by passive diffusion throughout the small intestine.
- Sodium Bicarbonate is absorbed by active transport and glucose and amino acid co-transport.
- Fructose is absorbed by facilitated diffusion.

Conditions Affecting the Small Intestine

The small intestine is a complex organ, and as such, there are a very large number of possible conditions that may affect the function of the small bowel. A few of them are listed below, some of which are common, with up to 10% of people being affected at some time in their lives, while others are vanishingly rare.

- Small intestine obstruction or obstructive disorders
  - Paralytic ileus
  - Volvulus
  - Hernia
  - Adhesions
  - Obstruction from external pressure
  - Obstruction by masses in the lumen (foreign bodies, bezoar, gallstones)
- Infectious diseases
  - Giardiasis
  - Ascariasis
  - Tropical sprue
  - Tape worm (Diphyllobothrium latum, Taenia Solium, Taenia solium, Hymenolepsis nana)
  - Hookworm (e.g. Necator americanus, Ancylostoma duodenale)
  - Nematodes (e.g. Ascaris lumbricoides)
  - Other Protozoa (e.g. Cryptosporidium parvum, Isopora belli, Cyclospora, Microsporidia, Entamoeba histolytica)
  - Bacterial Infections
    - Enterotoxigenic E. coli
    - Salmonella enterica
    - Campylobacter
    - Shigella
    - Yersinia
    - Clostridium difficile (antibiotic-associated colitis, Pseudomembranous Colitis
    - Mycobacterium (disseminated Mycobacterium tuberculosis)
    - Whipple's Disease
    - Vibrio (Cholera
    - Enteric (Typhoid) Fever (Salmonella enterica var. typhii) and Paratyphoid fever
    - Bacillus cereus
    - Clostridium perfringens (Gas Gangrene)
  - Viral Infections
    - Rotavirus
    - Norovirus
    - Astrovirus
    - Adenovirus
    - Calicivirus
  - Small bowel bacterial overgrowth syndrome
- Neoplasms (Cancers)
  - Adenocarcinoma
  - Carcinoid
  - Gastrointestinal Stromal Tumor (GIST)
  - Lymphoma

    - Sarcoma
    - Leiomyoma
    - metastatic tumors, especially SCLC or Melanoma
- Developmental, Congenital or Genetic Conditions
    - Duodenal (Intestinal) Atresia
    - Hirschsprung's Disease
    - Meckel's Diverticulum
    - Pyloric Stenosis
    - Pancreas Divisum
    - Ectopic Pancreas
    - Enteric duplication cyst
    - Situs Inversus
    - Cystic Fibrosis
    - Malrotation
    - Persistent Urachus
    - Omphalocele
    - Gastroschisis
    - Disachharidase (lactase) deficiencies
    - Primary Bile Acid Malsorption
    - Gardner Syndrome
    - Familial Adenomatous Polyposis Syndrome (FAP)
- Other Conditions
    - Crohn's disease, and the more general Inflammatory Bowel Disease
    - Typhlitis (neutropenic colitis in the immunosuppressed
    - Celiac disease (Sprue or Non-Tropical Sprue)
    - Mesenteric ischemia
    - Embolus or Thrombus of the Superior Mesenteric Artery or the Superior Mesenteric Vein
    - Arteriovenous malformation
    - Gastric dumping syndrome
    - Irritable Bowel Syndrome
    - Duodenal (Peptic) Ulcers
    - Gastrointestinal Perforation
    - Lymphatic Obstruction due to various causes
    - Hyperthyroidism
    - Diabetic Neuropathy
    - Diverticula
    - Radiation Enterocolitis
    - Drug Induced Injury
    - Diversion Colitis
    - Mesenteric Cysts
    - Peritoneal Infection
    - Sclerosing Retroperitonitis

In other animals

The small intestine is found in all tetrapods and also in teleosts, although its form and length vary enormously between species. In teleosts, it is relatively short, typically around one and a half times the length of the fish's body. It commonly has a number of *pyloric caeca*, small pouch-like structures along its length that help to increase the overall surface area of the organ for digesting food. There is no ileocaecal valve in teleosts, with the boundary between the small intestine and the rectum being marked only by the end of the digestive epithelium.[8]

In tetrapods, the ileocaecal valve is always present, opening into the colon. The length of the small intestine is typically longer in tetrapods than in teleosts, but is especially so in herbivores, as well as in mammals and birds, which have a higher metabolic rate than amphibians or reptiles. The lining of the small intestine includes microscopic folds to increase its surface area in all vertebrates, but only in mammals do these develop into true villi.[8]

The boundaries between the duodenum, jejunum, and ileum are somewhat vague even in humans, and such distinctions are either ignored when discussing the anatomy of other animals, or are essentially arbitrary.[8]

There is no small intestine as such in non-teleost fish, such as sharks, sturgeons, and lungfish. Instead, the digestive part of the gut forms a **spiral intestine**, connecting the stomach to the rectum. In this type of gut, the intestine itself is relatively straight, but has a long fold running along the inner surface in a spiral fashion, sometimes for dozens of turns. This valve greatly increases both the surface area and the effective length of the intestine. The lining of the spiral intestine is similar to that of the small intestine in teleosts and non-mammalian tetrapods.[8]

In lampreys, the spiral valve is extremely small, possibly because their diet requires little digestion. Hagfish have no spiral valve at all, with digestion occurring for almost the entire length of the intestine, which is not subdivided into different regions.[8]

References

- Sherwood, Lauralee (2006). *Fundamentals of physiology: a human perspective* [9] (Third ed.). Florence, KY: Cengage Learning. pp. 768. ISBN 0-53-446697-4.
- Solomon et al. (2002) Biology Sixth Edition, Brooks-Cole/Thomson Learning ISBN 0-03-033503-5
- Townsend et al. (2004) Sabiston Textbook of Surgery, Elsevier ISBN 0-7216-0409-9
- Thomson A, Drozdowski L, Iordache C, Thomson B, Vermeire S, Clandinin M, Wild G (2003). "Small bowel review: Normal physiology, part 1.". *Dig Dis Sci* **48** (8): 1546–64. doi:10.1023/A:1024719925058. PMID 12924651.
- Thomson A, Drozdowski L, Iordache C, Thomson B, Vermeire S, Clandinin M, Wild G (2003). "Small bowel review: Normal physiology, part 2.". *Dig Dis Sci* **48** (8): 1565–81. doi:10.1023/A:1024724109128. PMID 12924652.

Notes

[1] http://education.yahoo.com/reference/gray/subjects/subject?id=248#p1168
[3] http://www.nlm.nih.gov/cgi/mesh/2011/MB_cgi?mode=&term=Small+intestine
[4] http://www.mercksource.com/pp/us/cns/cns_hl_dorlands_split.jsp?pg=/ppdocs/us/common/dorlands/dorland/four/000054357.htm
[5] http://www.britannica.com/EBchecked/topic/275485/human-body
[6] "Elsevier: Gray's Anatomy, 40th Edition" (http://www.bartleby.com/107/248.html#txt168). .
[7] "Lea Brothers and Co. 1907: Surgical Applied Anatomy" (http://www.archive.org/stream/surgicalapplieda1907trev#page/n7/mode/2up).
.
[8] Romer, Alfred Sherwood; Parsons, Thomas S. (1977). *The Vertebrate Body*. Philadelphia, PA: Holt-Saunders International. pp. 349–353. ISBN 0-03-910284-X.
[9] http://books.google.com/?id=GoMD0tpYgBkC

Additional images

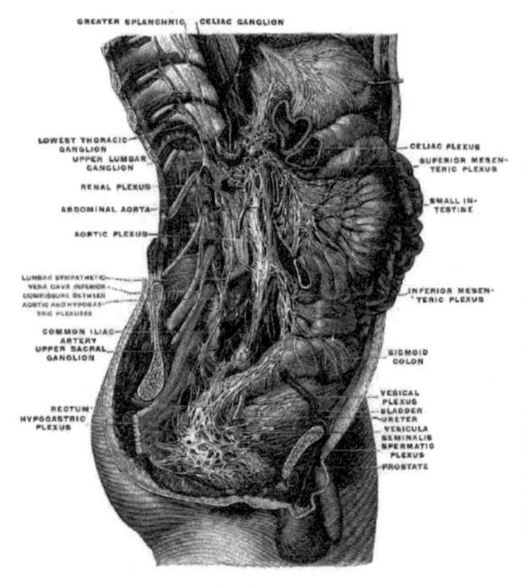

Lower half of right sympathetic cord.

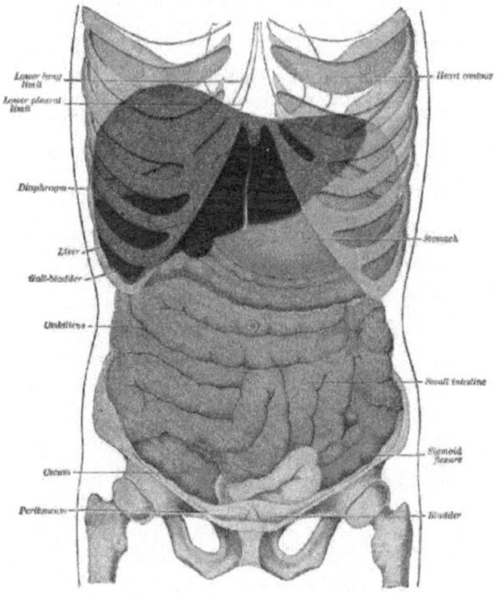

Topography of thoracic and abdominal viscera.

Large intestine

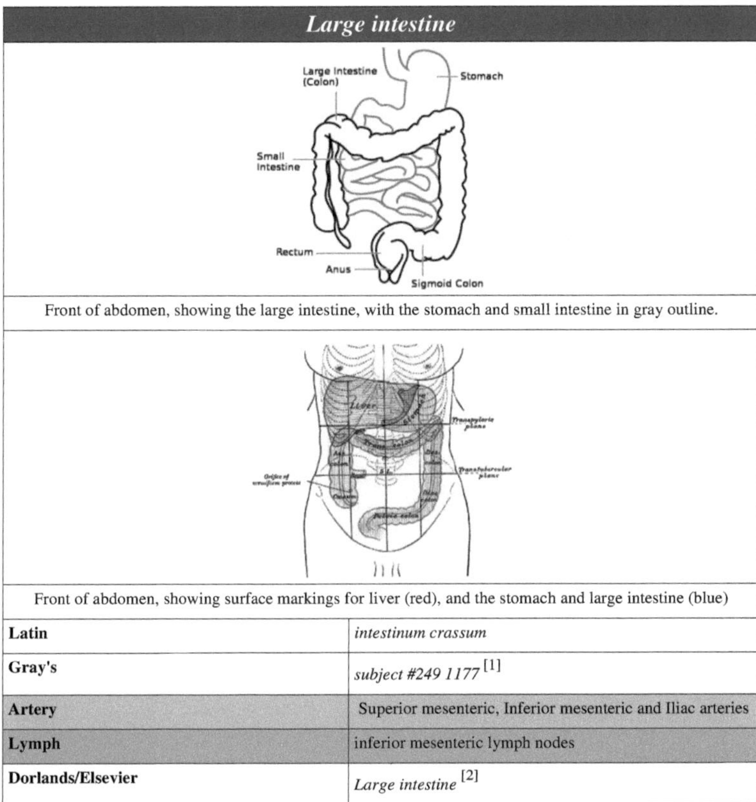

Large intestine	
Front of abdomen, showing the large intestine, with the stomach and small intestine in gray outline.	
Front of abdomen, showing surface markings for liver (red), and the stomach and large intestine (blue)	
Latin	*intestinum crassum*
Gray's	*subject #249 1177* [1]
Artery	Superior mesenteric, Inferior mesenteric and Iliac arteries
Lymph	inferior mesenteric lymph nodes
Dorlands/Elsevier	*Large intestine* [2]

The **large intestine** (or "large bowel") is the third-to-last part of the digestive system — — in vertebrate animals. Its function is to absorb water from the remaining indigestible food matter, and then to pass useless waste material from the body.[3] This article is primarily about the human gut, though the information about its processes are directly applicable to most mammals.

The large intestine consists of the cecum and colon. It starts in the right iliac region of the pelvis, just at or below the right waist, where it is joined to the bottom end of the small intestine. From here it continues up the abdomen, then across the width of the abdominal cavity, and then it turns down, continuing to its endpoint at the anus.

The large intestine is about 4.9 feet (1.5 m) long, which is about one-fifth of the whole length of the intestinal canal.

In Terminologia Anatomica the large intestine includes the cecum, colon, rectum, and anal canal. However, some sources exclude the anal canal.[4]

Function and relation to other organs

The large intestine takes about 16 hours to finish up the remaining processes of the digestive system. Food is no longer broken down at this stage of digestion. The colon absorbs vitamins which are created by the colonic bacteria - such as vitamin K (especially important as the daily ingestion of vitamin K is not normally enough to maintain adequate blood coagulation), vitamin B12, thiamine and riboflavin. It also compacts feces, and stores fecal matter in the rectum until it can be discharged via the anus in defecation.

The large intestine differs in physical form from the small intestine in being much wider and in showing the longitudinal layer of the muscularis have been reduced to 3 strap-like structures known as the taeniae coli. The wall of the large intestine is lined with simple columnar epithelium. Instead of having the evaginations of the small intestine (villi), the large intestine has invaginations (the intestinal glands). While both the small intestine and the large intestine have goblet cells, they are abundant in the large intestine.

The appendix is attached to its inferior surface of the cecum. It contains the least of lymphoid tissue. It is a part of mucosa-associated lymphoid tissue, which gives the appendix an important role in immunity. Appendicitis is the result of a blockage that traps infectious material in the lumen. The appendix can be removed with no apparent damage or consequence to the patient. The large intestine extends from the ileocecal junction to the anus and is about 4.9 ft long. On the surface, bands of longitudinal muscle fibers called taeniae coli, each about 1/5 in wide, can be identified. There are three bands, and they start at the base of the appendix and extend from the cecum to the rectum. Along the sides of the taeniae, tags of peritoneum filled with fat, called epiploic appendages (or appendices epiploicae) are found. The sacculations, called haustra, are characteristic features of the large intestine, and distinguish it from the small intestine.

Parts and location

Parts of the large intestine are:

Cecum – the first part of the large intestine

- Taeniae coli – three bands of smooth muscle
- Haustra – bulges caused by contraction of taeniae coli
- Epiploic appendages – small fat accumulations on the viscera

Locations along the colon are:

- The ascending colon
- The right colic flexure (hepatic)
- The transverse colon
- The transverse mesocolon
- The left colic flexure (splenic)
- The descending colon
- The sigmoid colon – the v-shaped region of the large intestine

Bacterial flora

The large intestine houses over 700 species of bacteria that perform a variety of functions.

The large intestine absorbs some of the products formed by the bacteria inhabiting this region. Undigested polysaccharides (fiber) are metabolized to short-chain fatty acids by bacteria in the large intestine and absorbed by passive diffusion. The bicarbonate that the large intestine secretes helps to neutralize the increased acidity resulting from the formation of these fatty acids.

These bacteria also produce large amounts of vitamins, especially vitamin K and biotin (a B vitamin), for absorption into the blood. Although this source of vitamins, in general, provides only a small part of the daily requirement, it makes a significant contribution when dietary vitamin intake is low. An individual that depends on absorption of vitamins formed by bacteria in the large intestine may become vitamin-deficient if treated with antibiotics that inhibit other species of bacteria as well as the disease-causing bacteria.

Other bacterial products include gas (flatus), which is a mixture of nitrogen and carbon dioxide, with small amounts of the gases hydrogen, methane, and hydrogen sulphide. Bacterial fermentation of undigested polysaccharides produces these. The normal flora is also essential in the development of certain tissues, including the cecum and lymphatics.

They are also involved in the production of cross-reactive antibodies. These are antibodies produced by the immune system against the normal flora, that are also effective against related pathogens, thereby preventing infection or invasion.

The most prevalent bacteria are the bacteroides, which have been implicated in the initiation of colitis and colon cancer. Bifidobacteria are also abundant, and are often described as 'friendly bacteria'.

A mucus layer protects the large intestine from attacks from colonic commensal bacteria.[5]

In other animals

The large intestine is truly distinct only in tetrapods, in which it is almost always separated from the small intestine by an ileocaecal valve. In most vertebrates, however, it is a relatively short structure running directly to the anus, although noticeably wider than the small intestine. Although the caecum is present in most amniotes, only in mammals does the remainder of the large intestine develop into a true colon.[6]

In some small mammals, the colon is straight, as it is in other tetrapods, but, in the majority of mammalian species, it is divided into ascending and descending portions; a distinct transverse colon is typically present only in primates. However, the taeniae coli and accompanying haustra are not found in either carnivorans or ruminants. The rectum of mammals (other than monotremes) is derived from the cloaca of other vertebrates, and is, therefore, not truly homologous with the "rectum" found in these species.[6]

In fish, there is no true large intestine, but simply a short rectum connecting the end of the digestive part of the gut to the cloaca. In sharks, this includes a *rectal gland* that secretes salt to help the animal maintain osmotic balance with the seawater. The gland somewhat resembles a caecum in structure, but is not a homologous structure.[6]

References

[1] http://education.yahoo.com/reference/gray/subjects/subject?id=249#p1177

[2] http://www.mercksource.com/pp/us/cns/cns_hl_dorlands_split.jsp?pg=/ppdocs/us/common/dorlands/dorland/four/000054354.htm

[3] Maton, Anthea; Jean Hopkins, Charles William McLaughlin, Susan Johnsons, Maryanna Quon Warner, David LaHart, Jill D. Wright (1993). *Human Biology and Health*. Englewood Cliffs, New Jersey, USA: Prentice Hall. ISBN 0-13-981176-1.

[4] "Dorlands Medical Dictionary:large intestine" (http://www.mercksource.com/pp/us/cns/cns_hl_dorlands_split.jspzQzpgzEzzSzppdocszSzuszSzcommonzSzdorlandszSzdorlandzSzfourzSz000054354zPzhtm). . Retrieved 2010-08-24.

[5] Stremmel, W; Merle, U; Zahn, A; Autschbach, F; Hinz, U; Ehehalt, R (2005). "Retarded release phosphatidylcholine benefits patients with chronic active ulcerative colitis" (http://gut.bmj.com/cgi/content/full/54/7/966). *Gut* **54** (7): 966–971. doi:10.1136/gut.2004.052316. PMC 1774598. PMID 15951544. .

[6] Romer, Alfred Sherwood; Parsons, Thomas S. (1977). *The Vertebrate Body*. Philadelphia, PA: Holt-Saunders International. pp. 351–354. ISBN 0-03-910284-X.

External links

- Overview and diagrams at seer.cancer.gov (http://training.seer.cancer.gov/anatomy/digestive/regions/intestine.html)
- *09-118h.* (http://www.merck.com/mmhe/sec09/ch118/ch118h.html) at Merck Manual of Diagnosis and Therapy Home Edition
- Photo at mgccc.cc.ms.us (http://learning.mgccc.cc.ms.us/science/cat/sld021.htm)
- MeSH *Large+Intestine* (http://www.nlm.nih.gov/cgi/mesh/2011/MB_cgi?mode=&term=Large+Intestine)

This article was originally based on an entry from a public domain edition of Gray's Anatomy. *As such, some of the information contained within it may be outdated.*

Gastrointestinal physiology

Gastrointestinal physiology is a branch of human physiology addressing the physical function of the gastrointestinal (GI) system. The major processes occurring in the GI system are that of motility, secretion, regulation, digestion and circulation. The function and coordination of each of these actions is vital in maintaining GI health, and thus the digestion of nutrients for the entire body.

Motility

The GI tract generates motility using smooth muscle subunits linked by gap junctions. These subunits fire spontaneously in either a tonic or a phasic fashion. Tonic contractions are those contractions that are maintained from several minutes up to hours at a time. These occur in the sphincters of the tract, as well as in the anterior stomach. The other type of contractions, called phasic contractions, consist of brief periods of both relaxation and contraction, occurring in the posterior stomach and the small intestine, and are carried out by the muscularis externa.

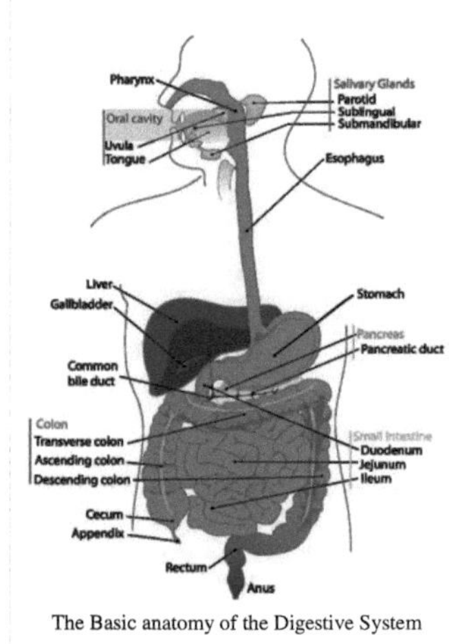

The Basic anatomy of the Digestive System

Stimulation

The stimulation for these contractions likely originates in modified smooth muscle cells called interstitial cells of Cajal. These cells cause spontaneous cycles of slow wave potentials that can cause action potentials in smooth muscle cells. They are associated with the contractile smooth muscle via gap junctions. These slow wave potentials must reach a threshold level for the action potential to occur, whereupon Ca^{2+} channels on the smooth muscle open and an action potential occurs. As the contraction is graded based upon how much Ca^{2+} enters the cell, the longer the duration of slow wave, the more action potentials occur. This in turn results in greater contraction force from the smooth muscle. Both amplitude and duration of the slow waves can be modified based upon the presence of neurotransmitters, hormones or other paracrine signaling. The number of slow wave potentials per minute varies based upon the location in the digestive tract. This number ranges from 3 waves/min in the stomach to 12 waves/min in the intestines.[1]

Contraction Patterns

The patterns of GI contraction as a whole can be divided into two distinct patterns, peristalsis and segmentation. Occurring between meals, the migrating motor complex is a series of peristaltic wave's cycles in distinct phases starting with relaxation followed by an increasing level of activity to a peak level of peristaltic activity lasting for 5–15 minutes.[2] This cycle repeats every 1.5–2 hours but is interrupted by food ingestion. The role of this process is likely to clean excess bacteria and food from the digestive system.[3]

Peristalsis

Peristalsis is the second of the three patterns and is one of the patterns that occur during and shortly after a meal. The contractions occur in wave patterns traveling down short lengths of the GI tract from one section to the next. The contractions occur directly behind the bolus of food that is in the system, forcing it toward the anus into the next relaxed section of smooth muscle. This relaxed section then contracts, generating smooth forward movement of the bolus at between 2–25 cm per second. This contraction pattern depends upon hormones, paracrine signals, and the autonomic nervous system for proper regulation.[1]

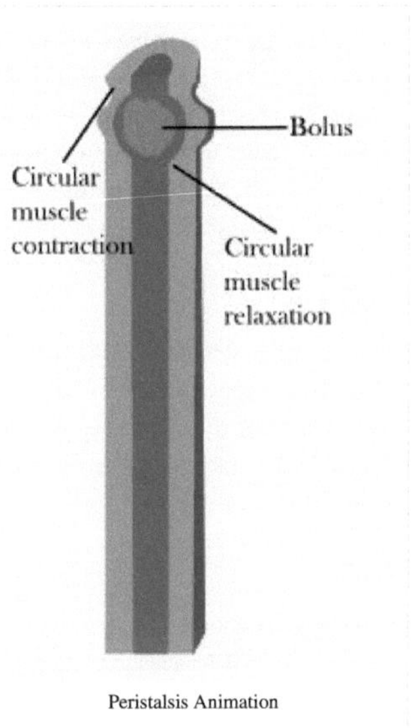

Peristalsis Animation

Segmentation

The third contraction pattern is segmentation, which also occurs during and shortly after a meal within short lengths in segmented or random patterns along the intestine. This process is carried out by longitudinal muscles relaxing while circular muscles contract at alternating sections thereby mixing the food. This mixing allows food and digestive enzymes to maintain a uniform composition, as well as to ensure contact with the epithelium for proper absorption.[1]

Secretion

Every day, seven liters of fluid are secreted by the digestive system. This fluid is composed of four primary components: ions, digestive enzymes, mucus, and bile. About half of these fluids are secreted by the salivary glands, pancreas, and liver, which compose the accessory organs and glands of the digestive system. The rest of the fluid is secreted by the GI epithelial cells.

Ions

The largest component of secreted fluids is ions and water, which are first secreted and then reabsorbed along the tract. The ions secreted primarily consist of H+, K+, Cl-, HCO3- and Na+. Water follows the movement of these ions. The GI tract accomplishes this ion pumping using a system of proteins that are capable of active transport, facilitated diffusion and open channel ion movement. The arrangement of these proteins on the apical and basolateral sides of the epithelium determines the net movement of ions and water in the tract.

H+ and Cl- are secreted by the parietal cells into the lumen of the stomach creating acidic conditions with a low pH of 1. H+ is pumped into the stomach by exchanging it with K+. This process also requires ATP as a source of energy; however, Cl- then follows the positive charge in the H+ through an open apical channel protein.

HCO_3^- secretion occurs to neutralize the acid secretions that make their way into the duodenum of the small intestine. Most of the HCO_3^- comes from pancreatic acinar cells in the form of $NaHCO_3$ in a watery solution.[2] This is the result of the high concentration of both HCO_3^- and Na^+ present in the duct creating an osmotic gradient to which the water follows.[1]

Digestive Enzymes

The second vital secretion of the GI tract is that of digestive enzymes that are secreted in the mouth, stomach and intestines. Some of these enzymes are secreted by accessory digestive organs, while others are secreted by the epithelial cells of the stomach and intestine. While some of these enzymes remain embedded in the wall of the GI tract, others are secreted in an inactive proenzyme form.[1] When these proenzymes reach the lumen of the tract, a factor specific to a particular proenzyme will activate it. A prime example of this is pepsin, which is secreted in the stomach by chief cells. Pepsin in its secreted form is inactive (pepsinogen). However, once it reaches the gastic lumen it becomes activated into pepsin by the high H^+ concentration, becoming an enzyme vital to digestion. The release of the enzymes is regulated by neural, hormonal, or paracrine signals. However, in general, parasympathetic stimulation increases secretion of all digestive enzymes.

Mucus

Mucus is released in the stomach and intestine, and serves to lubricate and protect the inner mucosa of the tract. It is composed of a specific family of glycoproteins termed mucins and is generally very viscous. Mucus is made by two types of specialized cells termed mucus cells in the stomach and goblet cells in the intestines. Signals for increased mucus release include parasympathetic innervations, immune system response and enteric nervous system messengers.[1]

Bile

Bile is secreted into the duodenum of the small intestine via the common bile duct. It is produced in liver cells and stored in the gall bladder until release during a meal. Bile is formed of three elements: bile salts, bilirubin and cholesterol. Bilirubin is a waste product of the breakdown of hemoglobin. The cholesterol present is secreted with the feces. The bile salt component is an active non-enzymatic substance that facilitates fat absorption by helping it to form an emulsion with water due to its amphoteric nature. These salts are formed in the hepatocytes from bile acids combined with an amino acid. Other compounds such as the waste products of drug degradation are also present in the bile.[2]

Regulation

The digestive system has a complex system of motility and secretion regulation which is vital for proper function. This task is accomplished via a system of long reflexes from the central nervous system (CNS), short reflexes from the enteric nervous system (ENS) and reflexes from GI peptides working in harmony with each other.[1]

Long Reflexes

Long reflexes to the digestive system involve a sensory neuron sending information to the brain, which integrates the signal and then sends messages to the digestive system. While in some situations, the sensory information comes from the GI tract itself; in others, information is received from sources other than the GI tract. When the latter situation occurs, these reflexes are called feedforward reflexes. This type of reflex includes reactions to food or danger triggering effects in the GI tract. Emotional responses can also trigger GI response such as the butterflies in the stomach feeling when nervous. The feedforward and emotional reflexes of the GI tract are considered cephalic reflexes.[1]

Short Reflexes

Control of the digestive system is also maintained by ENS, which can be thought of as a digestive brain that can help to regulate motility, secretion and growth. Sensory information from the digestive system can be received, integrated and acted upon by the enteric system alone. When this occurs, the reflex is called a short reflex.[1] Although this may be the case in several situations, the ENS can also work in conjunction with the CNS; vagal afferents from the viscera are received by the medulla, efferents are effected by the vagus nerve. When this occurs, the reflex is called vagovagal reflex. The Myenteric plexus and Submucosal plexus are both located in the gut wall and receive sensory signals from the lumen of the gut or the CNS.[2]

GI Peptides

GI peptides are signal molecules that are released into the blood by the GI cells themselves. They act on a variety of tissues including the brain, digestive accessory organs, and the GI tract. The effects range from excitatory or inhibitory effects on motility and secretion to feelings of satiety or hunger when acting on the brain. These hormones fall into three major categories, the gastrin and secretin families, with the third composed of all the other hormones unlike those in the other two families. Further information on the GI peptides is summarized in the table below.[3]

General GI Peptide Information

	Secreted By	Target	Effects on Endocrine Secretion	Effects on Exocrine Secretion	Effects on Motility	Other Effects	Stimulus for Release
Gastrin	G Cells in stomach	ECL cells; parietal cells	None	Increases acid secretion, increases mucus growth	None	None	Peptides and amino acids in lumen; gastrin releasing peptide and Ach in nervous reflexes
Cholecystokinin (CCK)	Endocrine cells of the small intestine; neurons of the brain and gut	Gallbladder, pancreas, gastric smooth muscle	None	Stimulates pancreatic enzyme and HCO3- secretion	Stimulates gallbladder contraction; Inhibits stomach emptying	Satiety	Fatty Acids and some Amino acids
Secretin	Endocrine Cells of the Small Intestine	Pancreas, stomach	None	Stimulates pancreatic and hepatic HCO3- secretion; Inhibits acid secretion; Pancreatic growth	Stimulates gallbladder contraction; Inhibits stomach emptying	None	Acid in small intestine
Gastric inhibitory Peptide	Endocrine K Cells of the small intestine	Beta Cells of the pancreas	Stimulates pancreatic insulin release	Inhibits Acid Secretion	None	Satiety and lipid metabolism	Glucose, Fatty Acid, and amino acids in small intestine
Motilin	Endocrine Cells in Small intestine	Smooth muscle of antrum and duodenum	None	None	Stimulates Migrating motor complex	Action in Brain?, Stimulates Migratory Motor Complex	Fasting: Cyclic release every 1.5–2 hours by neural stimulus.

Glucagon Like Peptide 1	Endocrine Cells in Small Intestine	Endocrine Pancreas	Stimulates Insulin release; inhibits glucagon release	Possibly Inhibits Acid Secretion	Slows gastric Emptying	Satiety	Mixed meals of Fats and Carbohydrates.

Digestion

- carbohydrates (monosaccharide, disaccharide)
- proteins
- lipids

Splanchnic circulation

- superior mesenteric artery
- inferior mesenteric artery

External links

- Overview [4] at McGill University
- Overview [5] at Medical College of Georgia
- Notes [6] at University of Bristol
- MeSH *Digestive+Physiology* [7]

References

[1] Silverthorn Ph. D, Dee Unglaub (April 2, 2006). *Human Physiology: An Integrated Approach*. Benjamin Cummings. ISBN 0805368515.
[2] Bowen DVM PhD, R (July 5, 2006). "Pathophysiology of the Digestive System" (http://www.vivo.colostate.edu/hbooks/pathphys/digestion/index.html). . Retrieved 2008-03-19.
[3] Nosek PhD, T.M.. "Essentials Of Human Phyisology" (http://www.lib.mcg.edu/edu/eshuphysio/program/section6/6outline.htm). . Retrieved 2008-03-19.
[4] http://sprojects.mmi.mcgill.ca/giphysio/about.htm
[5] http://www.lib.mcg.edu/edu/eshuphysio/program/section6/6outline.htm
[6] http://www.bris.ac.uk/Depts/Physiology/Staff/LFD/text/dental-1GI.html
[7] http://www.nlm.nih.gov/cgi/mesh/2011/MB_cgi?mode=&term=Digestive+Physiology

Digestion

Digestion is the mechanical and chemical breakdown of food into smaller components that are more easily absorbed into a blood stream, for instance. Digestion is a form of catabolism: a breakdown of large food molecules to smaller ones.

In mammals, food enters the mouth, being chewed by teeth, with chemical processing beginning with chemicals in the saliva from the salivary glands. This is called mastication. Then it travels down the esophagus into the stomach, where hydrochloric acid kills most contaminating microorganisms and begins break down of some food (e.g., denaturation of protein), and chemical alteration of some. The hydrochloric acid has a low pH, which allows enzymes to work more efficiently. After some time (typically an hour or two in humans, 4–6 hours in dogs, somewhat shorter duration in house cats, ...), the resulting thick liquid is called chyme. Chyme will go through the small intestine, where 95% of absorption of nutrients occurs, through the large intestine with waste material eventually being eliminated during defecation.[1]

Other organisms use different mechanisms to digest food.

Digestive systems

Digestive systems take many, many forms. There is a fundamental distinction between internal and external digestion. External digestion was the first to evolve, and most fungi still rely on it.[2] In this process, enzymes are secreted into the environment surrounding the organism, where they break down an organic material, and some of the products diffuse back to the organism. Later, animals evolved by rolling into a tube and acquiring internal digestion, which is more efficient because more of the broken down products can be captured, and the chemical environment can be more efficiently controlled.[3]

Some organisms, including nearly all spiders, simply secrete biotoxins and digestive chemicals (e.g., enzymes) into the extracellular environment prior to ingestion of the consequent "soup". In others, once potential nutrients or food is inside the organism, digestion can be conducted to a vesicle or a sac-like structure, through a tube, or through several specialized organs aimed at making the absorption of nutrients more efficient.

Secretion systems

Bacteria use several systems to obtain nutrients from other organisms in the environments.

Channel transport system

In a channel transport system several proteins form a contiguous channel traversing the inner and outer membranes of the bacteria. It is a simple system, which consists of only three protein subunits: the ABC protein, membrane fusion protein (MFP), and outer membrane protein (OMP). This secretion system transports various molecules, from ions, drugs, to proteins of various sizes (20 - 900 kDa). The molecules secreted vary in size from the small *Escherichia coli* peptide colicin V, (10 kDa) to the *Pseudomonas fluorescens* cell adhesion protein LapA of 900 kDa.[4]

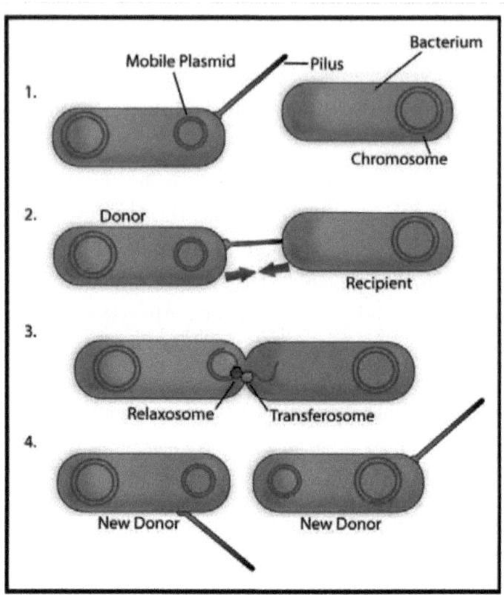

Schematic drawing of bacterial conjugation. **1-** Donor cell produces pilus. **2-** Pilus attaches to recipient cell, bringing the two cells together. **3-** The mobile plasmid is nicked and a single strand of DNA is transferred to the recipient cell. **4-** Both cells recircularize their plasmids, synthesize second strands, and reproduce pili; both cells are now viable donors.

Molecular syringe

One molecular syringe is used through which a bacterium (e.g. certain types of *Salmonella*, *Shigella*, *Yersinia*) can inject nutrients into protist cells. One such mechanism was first discovered in *Y. pestis* and showed that toxins could be injected directly from the bacterial cytoplasm into the cytoplasm of its host's cells rather than simply be secreted into the extracellular medium.[5]

Conjugation machinery

The conjugation machinery of some bacteria (and archaeal flagella) is capable of transporting both DNA and proteins. It was discovered in *Agrobacterium tumefaciens*, which uses this system to introduce the Ti plasmid and proteins into the host, which develops the crown gall (tumor).[6] The VirB complex of *Agrobacterium tumefaciens* is the prototypic system.[7]

The nitrogen fixing *Rhizobia* are an interesting case, wherein conjugative elements naturally engage in inter-kingdom conjugation. Such elements as the *Agrobacterium* Ti or Ri plasmids contain elements that can transfer to plant cells. Transferred genes enter the plant cell nucleus and effectively transform the plant cells into factories for the production of opines, which the bacteria use as carbon and energy sources. Infected plant cells form crown gall or root tumors. The Ti and Ri plasmids are thus endosymbionts of the bacteria, which are in turn endosymbionts (or parasites) of the infected plant.

The Ti and Ri plasmids are themselves conjugative. Ti and Ri transfer between bacteria uses an independent system (the *tra*, or transfer, operon) from that for inter-kingdom transfer (the *vir*, or virulence, operon). Such transfer creates virulent strains from previously avirulent *Agrobacteria*.

Release of outer membrane vesicles

In addition to the use of the multiprotein complexes listed above, Gram-negative bacteria possess another method for release of material: the formation of outer membrane vesicles.[8] Portions of the outer membrane pinch off, forming spherical structures made of a lipid bilayer enclosing periplasmic materials. Vesicles from a number of bacterial species have been found to contain virulence factors, some have immunomodulatory effects, and some can directly adhere to and intoxicate host cells. While release of vesicles has been demonstrated as a general response to stress conditions, the process of loading cargo proteins seems to be selective.[9]

Gastrovascular cavity

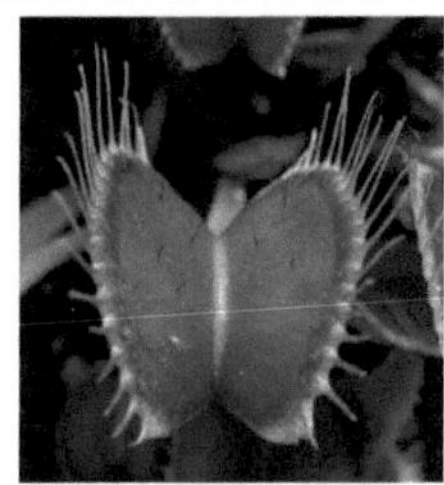

Venus Flytrap (*Dionaea muscipula*) leaf

The gastrovascular cavity functions as a stomach in both digestion and the distribution of nutrients to all parts of the body. Extracellular digestion takes place within this central cavity, which is lined with the gastrodermis, the internal layer of epithelium. This cavity has only one opening to the outside that functions as both a mouth and an anus: waste and undigested matter is excreted through the mouth/anus, which can be described as an incomplete gut.

In a plant such as the Venus Flytrap that can make its own food through photosynthesis, it does not eat and digest its prey for the traditional objectives of harvesting energy and carbon, but mines prey primarily for essential nutrients (nitrogen and phosphorus in particular) that are in short supply in its boggy, acidic habitat.[10]

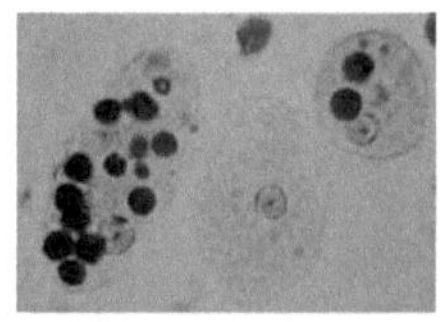

Trophozoites of *Entamoeba histolytica* with ingested erythrocytes

Phagosome

A phagosome is a vacuole formed around a particle absorbed by phagocytosis. The vacuole is formed by the fusion of the cell membrane around the particle. A phagosome is a cellular compartment in which pathogenic microorganisms can be killed and digested. Phagosomes fuse with lysosomes in their maturation process, forming phagolysosomes. In humans, *Entamoeba histolytica* can phagocytose red blood cells.[11]

Specialized organs and behaviors

To aid in the digestion of their food animals evolved organs such as beaks, tongues, teeth, a crop, gizzard, and others.

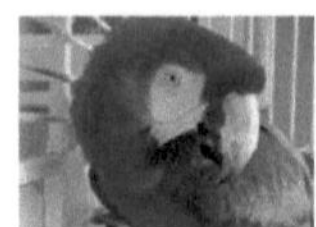

A Catalina Macaw's seed-shearing beak

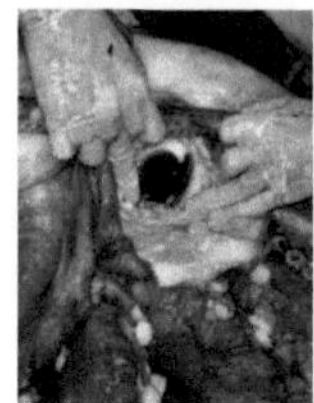

Squid beak with ruler for size comparison

Beaks

Macaws primarily eat seeds, nuts, and fruit, using their impressive beaks to open even the toughest seed. First they scratch a thin line with the sharp point of the beak, then they shear the seed open with the sides of the beak.

The mouth of the squid is equipped with a sharp horny beak mainly made of chitin[12] and cross-linked proteins. It is used to kill and tear prey into manageable pieces. The beak is very robust, but does not contain any minerals, unlike the teeth and jaws of many other organisms, including marine species.[13] The beak is the only indigestible part of the squid.

Tongue

The **tongue** is skeletal muscle on the floor of the mouth that manipulates food for chewing (mastication) and swallowing (deglutition). It is sensitive and kept moist by saliva. The underside of the tongue is covered with a smooth mucous membrane. The tongue is utilised to roll food particles into a bolus before being transported down the esophagus through the use of peristalsis. The sublingual region underneath the front of the tongue is a location where the oral mucosa is very thin, and underlain by a plexus of veins. This is an ideal location for introducing certain medications to the body. The sublingual route takes advantage of the highly vascular quality of the oral cavity, and allows for the speedy application of medication into the cardiovascular system, bypassing the gastrointestinal tract.

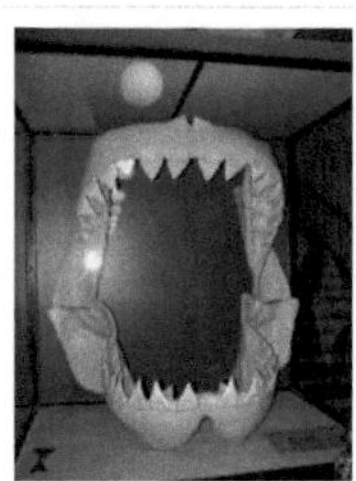

Teeth of a *Carcharodon megalodon*

Teeth

Teeth (singular, tooth) are small whitish structures found in the jaws (or mouths) of many vertebrates that are used to tear, scrape, milk and chew food. Teeth are not made of bone, but rather of tissues of varying density and hardness. The shape of an animal's teeth is related to its diet. For example, plant matter is hard to digest, so herbivores have many molars for chewing.

The teeth of carnivores are shaped to kill and tear meat, using specially shaped canine teeth. Herbivores' teeth are made for grinding food materials, in this case, plant parts.

Crop

A crop, or croup, is a thin-walled expanded portion of the alimentary tract used for the storage of food prior to digestion. In some birds it is an expanded, muscular pouch near the gullet or throat. In adult doves and pigeons, the crop can produce crop milk to feed newly hatched birds.[14]

Certain insects may have a crop or enlarged esophagus.

Abomasum

Herbivores have evolved cecums (or an abomasum in the case of ruminants). Ruminants have a fore-stomach with four chambers. These are the rumen, reticulum, omasum, and abomasum. In the first two chambers, the rumen and the reticulum, the food is mixed with saliva and separates into layers of solid and liquid material. Solids clump together to form the cud (or bolus). The cud is then regurgitated, chewed slowly to completely mix it with saliva and to break down the particle size.

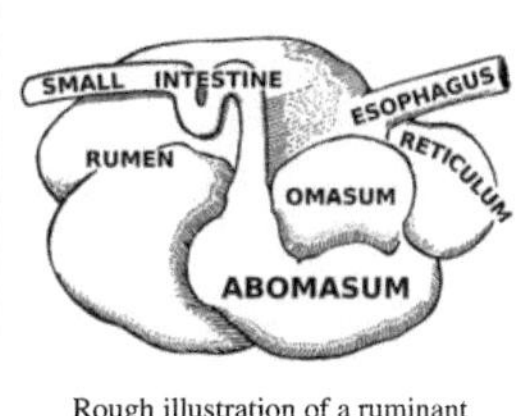

Rough illustration of a ruminant digestive system

Fiber, especially cellulose and hemi-cellulose, is primarily broken down into the volatile fatty acids, acetic acid, propionic acid and butyric acid in these chambers (the reticulo-rumen) by microbes: (bacteria, protozoa, and fungi). In the omasum water and many of the inorganic mineral elements are absorbed into the blood stream.

The abomasum is the fourth and final stomach compartment in ruminants. It is a close equivalent of a monogastric stomach (e.g., those in humans or pigs), and digesta is processed here in much the same way. It serves primarily as a site for acid hydrolysis of microbial and dietary protein, preparing these protein sources for further digestion and absorption in the small intestine. Digesta is finally moved into the small intestine, where the digestion and absorption of nutrients occurs. Microbes produced in the reticulo-rumen are also digested in the small intestine.

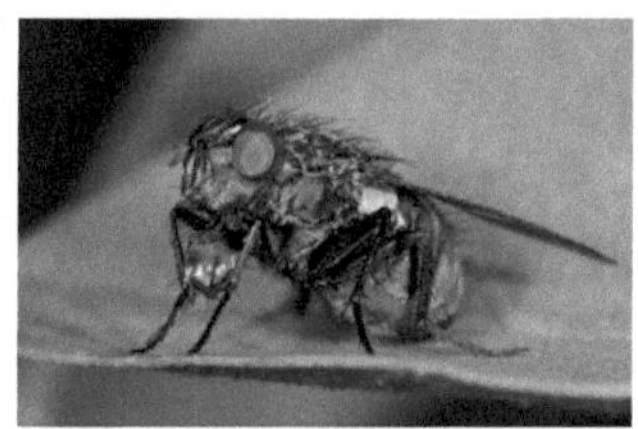
A flesh fly "blowing a bubble", possibly to concentrate its food by evaporating water

Specialized behaviors

Regurgitation has been mentioned above under abomasum and crop, referring to crop milk, a secretion from the lining of the crop of pigeons and doves with which the parents feed their young by regurgitation.[15]

Many sharks have the ability to turn their stomachs inside out and evert it out of their mouths in order to get rid of unwanted contents (perhaps developed as a way to reduce exposure to toxins).

Other animals, such as rabbits and rodents, practice coprophagia behaviors - eating specialized feces in order to re-digest food, especially in the case of roughage. Capybara, rabbits, hamsters and other related species do not have a complex digestive system as do, for example, ruminants. Instead they extract more nutrition from grass by giving their food a second pass through the gut. Soft fecal pellets of partially digested food are excreted and generally consumed immediately. They also produce normal droppings, which are not eaten.

Young elephants, pandas, koalas, and hippos eat the feces of their mother, probably to obtain the bacteria required to properly digest vegetation. When they are born, their intestines do not contain these bacteria (they are completely sterile). Without them, they would be unable to get any nutritional value from many plant components.

In earthworms

An earthworm's digestive system consists of a mouth, pharynx, esophagus, crop, gizzard, and intestine. The mouth is surrounded by strong lips, which act like a hand to grab pieces of dead grass, leaves, and weeds, with bits of soil to help chew. The lips break the food down into smaller pieces. In the pharynx the food is lubricated by mucus secretions for easier passage. The esophagus adds calcium carbonate to neutralize the acids formed by food matter decay. Temporary storage occurs in the crop where food and calcium carbonate are mixed. The powerful muscles of the gizzard churn and mix the mass of food and dirt. When the churning is complete, the glands in the walls of the gizzard add enzymes to the thick paste, which helps chemically breakdown the organic matter. By peristalsis the mixture is sent to the intestine where friendly bacteria continue chemical breakdown. This releases carbohydrates, protein, fat, and various vitamins and minerals for absorption into the body.

Overview of vertebrate digestion

In most vertebrates, digestion is a multi-stage process in the digestive system, starting from ingestion of raw materials, most often other organisms. Ingestion usually involves some type of mechanical and chemical processing. Digestion is separated into four steps:

1. Ingestion: placing food into the mouth (entry of food in the digestive system),
2. Mechanical and chemical breakdown: mastication and the mixing of the resulting bolus with water, acids, bile and enzymes in the stomach and intestine to break down complex molecules into simple structures,
3. Absorption: of nutrients from the digestive system to the circulatory and lymphatic capillaries through osmosis, active transport, and diffusion, and
4. Egestion (Excretion): Removal of undigested materials from the digestive tract through defecation.

Underlying the process is muscle movement throughout the system through swallowing and peristalsis. Each step in digestion requires energy, and thus imposes an "overhead charge" on the energy made available from absorbed substances. Differences in that overhead cost are important influences on lifestyle, behavior, and even physical structures. Examples may be seen in humans, who differ considerably from other hominids (lack of hair, smaller jaws and musculature, different dentition, length of intestines, cooking, etc.).

The major part of digestion takes place in the small intestine. The large intestine primarily serves as a site for fermentation of indigestible matter by gut bacteria and for resorption of water from digesta before excretion.

In mammals, preparation for digestion begins with the cephalic phase in which saliva is produced in the mouth and digestive enzymes are produced in the stomach. Mechanical and chemical digestion begin in the mouth where food is chewed, and mixed with saliva to begin enzymatic processing of starches. The stomach continues to break food down mechanically and chemically through churning and mixing with both acids and enzymes. Absorption occurs in the stomach and gastrointestinal tract, and the process finishes with defecation.[1]

Human digestion process

The whole digestive system is around 9 meters long. In a healthy human adult this process can take between 24 and 72 hours. Food digestion physiology varies between individuals and upon other factors such as the characteristics of the food and size of the meal.[16]

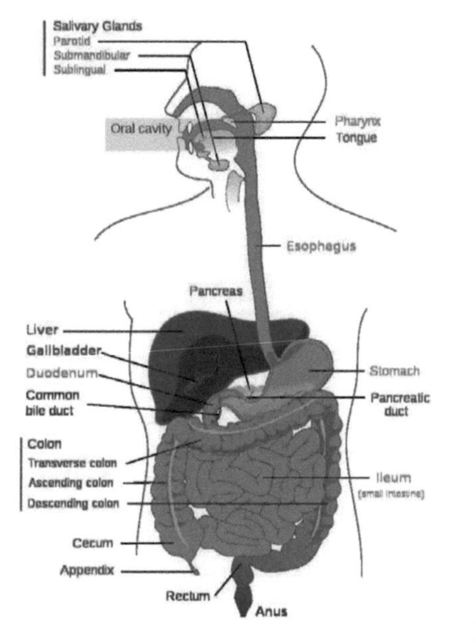

Upper and Lower human gastrointestinal tract

Phases of gastric secretion

- Cephalic phase - This phase occurs before food enters the stomach and involves preparation of the body for eating and digestion. Sight and thought stimulate the cerebral cortex. Taste and smell stimulus is sent to the hypothalamus and medulla oblongata. After this it is routed through the vagus nerve and release of acetylcholine. Gastric secretion at this phase rises to 40% of maximum rate. Acidity in the stomach is not buffered by food at this point and thus acts to inhibit parietal (secretes acid) and G cell (secretes gastrin) activity via D cell secretion of somatostatin.
- Gastric phase - This phase takes 3 to 4 hours. It is stimulated by distension of the stomach, presence of food in stomach and decrease in pH. Distention activates long and myenteric reflexes. This activates the release of acetylcholine, which stimulates the release of more gastric juices. As protein enters the stomach, it binds to hydrogen ions, which raises the pH of the stomach. Inhibition of gastrin and gastric acid secretion is lifted. This triggers G cells to release gastrin, which in turn stimulates parietal cells to secrete gastric acid. Gastric acid is about 0.5% hydrochloric acid (HCl), which lowers the pH to the desired pH of 1-3. Acid release is also triggered by acetylcholine and histamine.
- Intestinal phase - This phase has 2 parts, the excitatory and the inhibitory. Partially digested food fills the duodenum. This triggers intestinal gastrin to be released. Enterogastric reflex inhibits vagal nuclei, activating sympathetic fibers causing the pyloric sphincter to tighten to prevent more food from entering, and inhibits local reflexes.

Oral cavity

In humans, digestion begins in the oral cavity, otherwise known as the "Buccal Cavity", where food is chewed. Saliva is secreted in large amounts (1-1.5 litres/day) by three pairs of exocrine salivary glands (parotid, submandibular, and sublingual) in the oral cavity, and is mixed with the chewed food by the tongue. Saliva cleans the oral cavity, moistens the food, and contains digestive enzymes such as salivary amylase, which aids in the chemical breakdown of polysaccharides such as starch into disaccharides such as maltose. It also contains mucus, a glycoprotein that helps soften the food and form it into a bolus. An additional enzyme, lingual lipase, hydrolyzes long-chain triglycerides into partial glycerides and free fatty acids.

Swallowing transports the chewed food into the esophagus, passing through the oropharynx and hypopharynx. The mechanism for swallowing is coordinated by the swallowing center in the medulla oblongata and pons. The reflex is initiated by touch receptors in the pharynx as the bolus of food is pushed to the back of the mouth.

Pharynx

The pharynx is the part of the neck and throat situated immediately behind the mouth and nasal cavity, and cranial, or superior, to the esophagus. It is part of the digestive system and respiratory system. Because both food and air pass through the pharynx, a flap of connective tissue, the epiglottis closes over the trachea when food is swallowed to prevent choking or asphyxiation.

The oropharynx is that part of the pharynx behind the oral cavity. It is lined with stratified squamous epithelium. The nasopharynx lies behind the nasal cavity and like the nasal passages is lined with ciliated columnar pseudostratified epithelium.

Like the oropharynx above it the hypopharynx (laryngopharynx) serves as a passageway for food and air and is lined with a stratified squamous epithelium. It lies inferior to the upright epiglottis and extends to the larynx, where the respiratory and digestive pathways diverge. At that point, the laryngopharynx is continuous with the esophagus. During swallowing, food has the "right of way", and air passage temporarily stops.

Esophagus

The esophagus is a narrow muscular tube about 20-30 centimeters long, which starts at the pharynx at the back of the mouth, passes through the thoracic diaphragm, and ends at the cardiac orifice of the stomach. The wall of the esophagus is made up of two layers of smooth muscles, which form a continuous layer from the esophagus to the colon and contract slowly, over long periods of time. The inner layer of muscles is arranged circularly in a series of descending rings, while the outer layer is arranged longitudinally. At the top of the esophagus, is a flap of tissue called the epiglottis that closes during swallowing to prevent food from entering the trachea (windpipe). The chewed food is pushed down the esophagus to the stomach through peristaltic contraction of these muscles. It takes only about seven seconds for food to pass through the esophagus and now digestion takes place.

Stomach

The stomach is a small, 'J'-shaped pouch with walls made of thick, elastic muscles, which stores and helps break down food. Food reduced to very small particles is more likely to be fully digested in the small intestine, and stomach churning has the effect of assisting the physical disassembly begun in the mouth. Ruminants, who are able to digest fibrous material (primarily cellulose), use fore-stomachs and repeated chewing to further the disassembly. Rabbits and some other animals pass some material through their entire digestive systems twice. Most birds ingest small stones to assist in mechanical processing in gizzards.

Food enters the stomach through the cardiac orifice where it is further broken apart and thoroughly mixed with gastric acid, pepsin and other digestive enzymes to break down proteins. The enzymes in the stomach also have an optimum, meaning that they work at a specific pH and temperature better than any others. The acid itself does not break down food molecules, rather it provides an optimum pH for the reaction of the enzyme pepsin and kills many microorganisms that are ingested with the food. It can also denature proteins. This is the process of reducing polypeptide bonds and disrupting salt bridges, which in turn causes a loss of secondary, tertiary, or quaternary protein structure. The parietal cells of the stomach also secrete a glycoprotein called intrinsic factor, which enables the absorption of vitamin B-12. Mucus neck cells are present in the gastric glands of the stomach. They secrete mucus, which along with gastric juice plays and important role in lubrication and protection of the mucosal epithelium from excoriation by the highly concentrated hydrochloric acid. Other small molecules such as alcohol are absorbed in the stomach, passing through the membrane of the stomach and entering the circulatory system directly. Food in the stomach is in semi-liquid form, which upon completion is known as chyme.

After consumption of food, digestive "tonic" and peristaltic contractions begin, which helps break down the food and move it through.[16] When the chyme reaches the opening to the duodenum known as the pylorus, contractions "squirt" the food back into the stomach through a process called retropulsion, which exerts additional force and further grinds down food into smaller particles.[16] Gastric emptying is the release of food from the stomach into the duodenum; the process is tightly controlled with liquids being emptied much more quickly than solids.[16] Gastric emptying has attracted medical interest as rapid gastric emptying is related to obesity and delayed gastric emptying syndrome is associated with diabetes mellitus, aging, and gastroesophageal reflux.[16]

The transverse section of the alimentary canal reveals four (or five, see description under mucosa) distinct and well developed layers within the stomach:

- Serous membrane, a thin layer of mesothelial cells that is the outermost wall of the stomach.
- Muscular coat, a well-developed layer of muscles used to mix ingested food, composed of three sets running in three different alignments. The outermost layer runs parallel to the vertical axis of the stomach (from top to bottom), the middle is concentric to the axis (horizontally circling the stomach cavity) and the innermost oblique layer, which is responsible for mixing and breaking down ingested food, runs diagonal to the longitudinal axis. The inner layer is unique to the stomach, all other parts of the digestive tract have only the first two layers.
- Submucosa, composed of connective tissue that links the inner muscular layer to the mucosa and contains the nerves, blood and lymph vessels.
- Mucosa is the extensively folded innermost layer. It can be divided into the epithelium, lamina propria, and the muscularis mucosae, though some consider the outermost *muscularis mucosae* to be a distinct layer, as it develops from the mesoderm rather than the endoderm (thus making a total of five layers). The epithelium and lamina are filled with connective tissue and covered in gastric glands that may be simple or branched tubular, and secrete mucus, hydrochloric acid, pepsinogen and rennin. The mucus lubricates the food and also prevents hydrochloric acid from acting on the walls of the stomach.

Small intestine

It has three parts: the Duodenum, Jejunum, and Ileum.

After being processed in the stomach, food is passed to the small intestine via the pyloric sphincter. The majority of digestion and absorption occurs here after the milky chyme enters the duodenum. Here it is further mixed with three different liquids:

- Bile, which emulsifies fats to allow absorption, neutralizes the chyme and is used to excrete waste products such as bilin and bile acids. Bile is produced by the liver and then stored in the gallbladder. The bile in the gallbladder is much more concentrated.
- Pancreatic juice made by the pancreas.
- Intestinal enzymes of the alkaline mucosal membranes. The enzymes include maltase, lactase and sucrase (all three of which process only sugars), trypsin and chymotrypsin.

The pH level increases in the small intestine. A more basic environment causes more helpful enzymes to activate and begin to help in the breakdown of molecules such as fat globules. Small, finger-like structures called villi, each of which is covered with even smaller hair-like structures called microvilli improve the absorption of nutrients by increasing the surface area of the intestine and enhancing speed at which nutrients are absorbed. Blood containing the absorbed nutrients is carried away from the small intestine via the hepatic portal vein and goes to the liver for filtering, removal of toxins, and nutrient processing.

The small intestine and remainder of the digestive tract undergoes peristalsis to transport food from the stomach to the rectum and allow food to be mixed with the digestive juices and absorbed. The circular muscles and longitudinal muscles are antagonistic muscles, with one contracting as the other relaxes. When the circular muscles contract, the lumen becomes narrower and longer and the food is squeezed and pushed forward. When the longitudinal muscles contract, the circular muscles relax and the gut dilates to become wider and shorter to allow food to enter.

Large intestine

After the food has been passed through the small intestine, the food enters the large intestine. Within it, digestion is retained long enough to allow fermentation due to the action of gut bacteria, which breaks down some of the substances that remain after processing in the small intestine; some of the breakdown products are absorbed. In humans, these include most complex saccharides (at most three disaccharides are digestible in humans). In addition, in many vertebrates, the large intestine reabsorbs fluid; in a few, with desert lifestyles, this reabsorbtion makes continued existence possible.

In humans, the large intestine is roughly 1.5 meters long, with three parts: the cecum at the junction with the small intestine, the colon, and the rectum. The colon itself has four parts: the ascending colon, the transverse colon, the descending colon, and the sigmoid colon. The large intestine absorbs water from the bolus and stores feces until it can be egested. Food products that cannot go through the villi, such as cellulose (dietary fiber), are mixed with other waste products from the body and become hard and concentrated feces. The feces is stored in the rectum for a certain period and then the stored feces is eliminated from the body due to the contraction and relaxation through the anus. The exit of this waste material is regulated by the anal sphincter.

Breakdown into nutrients

Protein digestion

Protein digestion occurs in the stomach and duodenum in which 3 enzymes: pepsin secreted by the stomach and trypsin and chymotrypsin secreted by the pancreas breakdown food proteins into polypeptides that are then broken down by the enzyme erepsin into amino acids.

Fat digestion

Digestion of fat begins in the mouth where lingual lipase breaks down some lipids into diglycerides. The presence of fat in the small intestine produces hormones that stimulate the release of pancreatic lipase from the pancreas and bile from the liver for breakdown of fats into fatty acids.

Carbohydrate digestion

Starches are broken down into sugars (glucose and fructose) by amylase and hydrochloric acid in the stomach.

DNA and RNA digestion

DNA and RNA are broken down into mononucleotides by the nucleases deoxyribonuclease and ribonuclease (DNase and RNase) from the pancreas.

Digestive hormones

There are at least five hormones that aid and regulate the digestive system in mammals. There are variations across the vertebrates, as for instance in birds. Arrangements are complex and additional details are regularly discovered. For instance, more connections to metabolic control (largely the glucose-insulin system) have been uncovered in recent years.

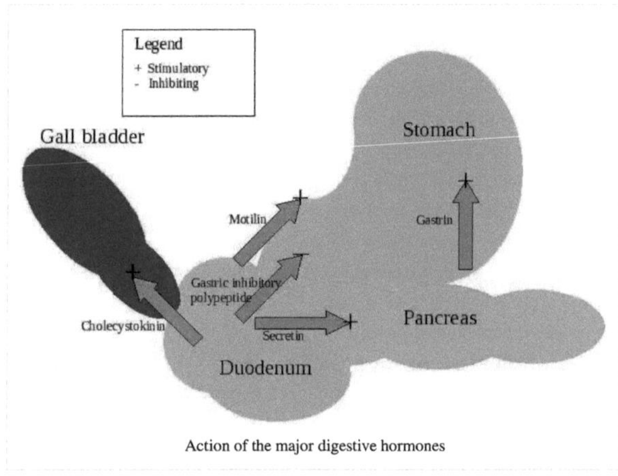

Action of the major digestive hormones

- Gastrin - is in the stomach and stimulates the gastric glands to secrete pepsinogen (an inactive form of the enzyme pepsin) and hydrochloric acid. Secretion of gastrin is stimulated by food arriving in stomach. The secretion is inhibited by low pH .
- Secretin - is in the duodenum and signals the secretion of sodium bicarbonate in the pancreas and it stimulates the bile secretion in the liver. This hormone responds to the acidity of the chyme.
- Cholecystokinin (CCK) - is in the duodenum and stimulates the release of digestive enzymes in the pancreas and stimulates the emptying of bile in the gall bladder. This hormone is secreted in response to fat in chyme.
- Gastric inhibitory peptide (GIP) - is in the duodenum and decreases the stomach churning in turn slowing the emptying in the stomach. Another function is to induce insulin secretion.
- Motilin - is in the duodenum and increases the migrating myoelectric complex component of gastrointestinal motility and stimulates the production of pepsin.

Significance of pH in digestion

Digestion is a complex process controlled by several factors. pH plays a crucial role in a normally functioning digestive tract. In the mouth, pharynx, and esophagus, pH is typically about 6.8, very weakly acidic. Saliva controls pH in this region of the digestive tract. Salivary amylase is contained in saliva and starts the breakdown of carbohydrates into monosaccharides. Most digestive enzymes are sensitive to pH and will denature in a high or low pH environment.

The stomach's high acidity inhibits the breakdown of carbohydrates within it. This acidity confers two benefits: it denatures proteins for further digestion in the small intestines, and provides non-specific immunity, damaging or eliminating various pathogens.

In the small intestines, the duodenum provides critical pH balancing to activate digestive enzymes. The liver secretes bile into the duodenum to neutralize the acidic conditions from the stomach, and the pancreatic duct empties into the duodenum, adding bicarbonate to neutralize the acidic chyme, thus creating a neutral environment. The mucosal tissue of the small intestines is alkaline with a pH of about 8.5.

Uses of animal gut by humans

- The stomachs of calves have commonly been used as a source of rennet for making cheese.
- The use of animal gut strings by musicians can be traced back to the third dynasty of Egypt. In the recent past, strings were made out of lamb gut. With the advent of the modern era, musicians have tended to use strings made of silk, or synthetic materials such as nylon or steel. Some instrumentalists, however, still use gut strings in order to evoke the older tone quality. Although such strings were commonly referred to as "catgut" strings, cats were never used as a source for gut strings.
- Sheep gut was the original source for natural gut string used in racquets, such as for tennis. Today, synthetic strings are much more common, but the best gut strings are now made out of cow gut.
- Gut cord has also been used to produce strings for the snares that provide a snare drum's characteristic buzzing timbre. While the modern snare drum almost always uses metal wire rather than gut cord, the North African bendir frame drum still uses gut for this purpose.
- "Natural" sausage hulls (or casings) are made of animal gut, especially hog, beef, and lamb. Similarly, Haggis is traditionally boiled in, and served in, a sheep stomach.
- Chitterlings, a kind of food, consist of thoroughly washed pig's gut.
- Animal gut was used to make the cord lines in longcase clocks and for fusee movements in bracket clocks, but may be replaced by metal wire.
- The oldest known condoms, from 1640 AD, were made from animal intestine.[17]

See also

- Nutrition
- Human gastrointestinal tract
- Stomach
- Gastroesophageal reflux disease
- Discovery and Development of Proton Pump Inhibitors

References

[1] Maton, Anthea; Jean Hopkins, Charles William McLaughlin, Susan Johnson, Maryanna Quon Warner, David LaHart, Jill D. Wright (1993). *Human Biology and Health*. Englewood Cliffs, New Jersey, USA: Prentice Hall. ISBN 0-13-981176-1. OCLC 32308337.

[2] Dusenbery, David B. (1996). "Life at Small Scale", pp. 113-115. Scientific American Library, New York. ISBN 0-7167-5060-0.

[3] Dusenbery, David B. (2009). *Living at Micro Scale*, p. 280. Harvard University Press, Cambridge, Mass. ISBN 978-0-674-03116-6.

[4] Wooldridge K (editor) (2009). *Bacterial Secreted Proteins: Secretory Mechanisms and Role in Pathogenesis*. Caister Academic Press. ISBN 978-1-904455-42-4.

[5] Salyers, A. A. & Whitt, D. D. (2002). *Bacterial Pathogenesis: A Molecular Approach*, 2nd ed., Washington, D.C.: ASM Press. ISBN 1-55581-171-X

[6] Cascales E & Christie P.J. (2003). "The versatile Type IV secretion systems". *Nat Rev Microbiol* **1** (2): 137–149. doi:10.1038/nrmicro753. PMID 15035043.

[7] Christie PJ, Atmakuri K, Jabubowski S, Krishnamoorthy V & Cascales E. (2005). "Biogenesis, architecture, and function of bacterial Type IV secretion systems". *Ann Rev Microbiol* **59**: 451–485. doi:10.1146/annurev.micro.58.030603.123630. PMID 16153176.

[8] Chatterjee, SN and J Das. "Electron microscopic observations on the excretion of cell wall material by *Vibrio cholerae*." "J.Gen.Microbiol." "49" : 1-11 (1967) ; Kuehn, MJ and NC Kesty. "Bacterial outer membrane vesicles and the host-pathogen interaction." *Genes Dev*.and then the **19**(22):2645-55 (2005)

[9] McBroom, AJ and MJ Kuehn Release of outer membrane vesicles by Gram-negative bacteria is a novel envelope stress response. (http://www.ncbi.nlm.nih.gov/pubmed/17163978) *Mol. Microbiol.* **63**(2):545-58 (2007)

[10] Leege, Lissa. "How does the Venus flytrap digest flies?" (http://www.sciam.com/article.cfm?id=how-does-the-venus-flytra). *Scientific American.* . Retrieved 2008-08-20.

[11] Boettner DR, Huston CD, Linford AS, *et al.* (January 2008). "Entamoeba histolytica phagocytosis of human erythrocytes involves PATMK, a member of the transmembrane kinase family" (http://www.plospathogens.org/article/info:doi/10.1371/journal.ppat.0040008). *PLoS Pathog.* **4** (1): e8. doi:10.1371/journal.ppat.0040008. PMC 2211552. PMID 18208324. .
[12] Clarke, M.R. (1986). *A Handbook for the Identification of Cephalopod Beaks.* Oxford: Clarendon Press. ISBN 0-19-857603-X.
[13] Miserez, A; Li, Y; Waite, H; Zok, F (2007). "Jumbo squid beaks: Inspiration for design of robust organic composites". *Acta Biomaterialia* **3** (1): 139–149. doi:10.1016/j.actbio.2006.09.004. PMID 17113369.
[14] Gordon John Larkman Ramel (2008-09-29). "The Alimentary Canal in Birds" (http://www.earthlife.net/birds/digestion.html). . Retrieved 2008-12-16.
[15] Levi, Wendell (1977). *The Pigeon.* Sumter, S.C.: Levi Publishing Co, Inc. ISBN 0853900132.
[16] Kong F, Singh RP (June 2008). "Disintegration of solid foods in human stomach". *J. Food Sci.* **73** (5): R67–80. doi:10.1111/j.1750-3841.2008.00766.x. PMID 18577009. Free full-text (http://onlinelibrary.wiley.com/doi/10.1111/j.1750-3841.2008.00766.x/full)
[17] "World's oldest condom" (http://www.ananova.com/news/story/sm_1870958.html?menu=news.quirkies.sexlife). Ananova. 2008. . Retrieved 2008-04-11.

External links

- Human Physiology - Digestion (http://homepage.ufp.pt/pedros/qfisio/digestion.htm)
- NIH guide to digestive system (http://digestive.niddk.nih.gov/ddiseases/pubs/yrdd/index.htm)
- The Digestive System (http://www.biology-innovation.co.uk/digestive_system.php)

Migrating motor complex

Migrating motor complexes (or **migrating myoelectric complex**) are waves of activity that sweep through the intestines in a regular cycle during fasting state.

These motor complexes help trigger peristaltic waves which facilitate transportation of indigestible substances such as bone, fiber and foreign bodies from the stomach, through the small intestine past the ileocecal sphincter into the colon.

The MMC originates in the stomach roughly every 75–90 minutes during the interdigestive phase (between meals) and is responsible for the rumbling experienced when hungry.

It also serves to transport bacteria from the small intestine to the large intestine, and to inhibit the migration of colonic bacteria into the terminal ileum.

The MMC is thought to be partially regulated by motilin which is initiated in the stomach as a response to vagal stimulation, and does not depend on extrinsic nerves directly.

References

- http://medical-dictionary.thefreedictionary.com/migrating+myoelectric+complex

External links

- Overview at colostate.edu [1]
- Physiology at MCG *6/6ch2/s6ch2_26* [2]
- MeSH *Migrating+motor+complex* [3]

References

[1] http://www.vivo.colostate.edu/hbooks/pathphys/digestion/stomach/mmcomplex.html
[2] http://www.lib.mcg.edu/edu/eshuphysio/program/section6/6ch2/s6ch2_26.htm
[3] http://www.nlm.nih.gov/cgi/mesh/2011/MB_cgi?mode=&term=Migrating+motor+complex

Borborygmus

Borborygmus (plural **borborygmi**, pronounced English pronunciation: /ˌbɔrbəˈrɪgməs/; from Greek *βορβορυγμός*) also known as **stomach growling, rumbling**, **gurgling**, **grumbling** or **wambling,** is the rumbling sound produced by the contraction of muscles in the stomach and intestines of animals, including humans.[1]

The "rumble" or "growl" sometimes heard from the stomach is a normal part of digestion. It originates in the stomach or upper part of the small intestine as muscles contract to move food and digestive juices down the gastrointestinal tract and functions as a sort of intestinal "housecleaning".[2] Sometimes it occurs as part of the migrating myoelectric complex.[3]

Although this muscle contraction happens whether or not food is present, it is more common after the animal has gone several hours without eating. This may be why a "growling" stomach is often associated with hunger.[3]

Rumbles may also occur when there is incomplete digestion of food that can lead to excess gas in the intestine. In humans this can be due to incomplete digestion of carbohydrate-containing foods including milk and other dairy products (lactose intolerance[2] or the use of α-glucosidase inhibitors by diabetics), gluten (protein in wheat, barley, and rye) (celiac disease), fruits, vegetables, beans, legumes, and high-fiber whole grains. In rare instances, excessive abdominal noise may be a sign of digestive disease, especially when accompanied by abdominal bloating, abdominal pain, diarrhea or constipation. Some examples of diseases that may be associated with this symptom include carcinoid neoplasm and celiac sprue.[2]

In the therapeutic theory and prectice of neo-Reichian therapist Gerda Boyesen borborygmus was termed *psychoperistalsis* and she linked it to the dynamics of the persons psychological processes.

Non-medical use

The word *borborygmic* has been used in literature to describe noisy plumbing. In *Ada*, Vladimir Nabokov wrote: "All the toilets and waterpipes in the house had been suddenly seized with borborygmic convulsions". In *A Long Way Down* (New York: Harper, 1959, p. 54), Elizabeth Fenwick wrote: "The room was very quiet, except for its borborygmic old radiator".[4]

See also

- Flatulence

References

[1] Dictionary entries for borborygmus (http://dictionary.reference.com/browse/borborygmus)
[2] Borborygmus – The Gurgling Intestines – Causes and Prevention (http://digestion.ygoy.com/borborygmus-the-gurgling-intestines-causes-and-prevention/)
[3] Why does your stomach growl when you are hungry? (http://www.scientificamerican.com/article.cfm?id=why-does-your-stomach-gro) Scientific American, January 21, 2002.
[4] BORBORYGMUS (http://www.worldwidewords.org/weirdwords/ww-bor1.htm) World Wide Words

Defecation

Defecation (from late Latin *defecatio*) is the final act of digestion by which organisms eliminate solid, semisolid or liquid waste material (feces) from the digestive tract via the anus. Waves of muscular contraction known as peristalsis in the walls of the colon move fecal matter through the digestive tract towards the rectum. Undigested food may also be expelled this way in the process called egestion.

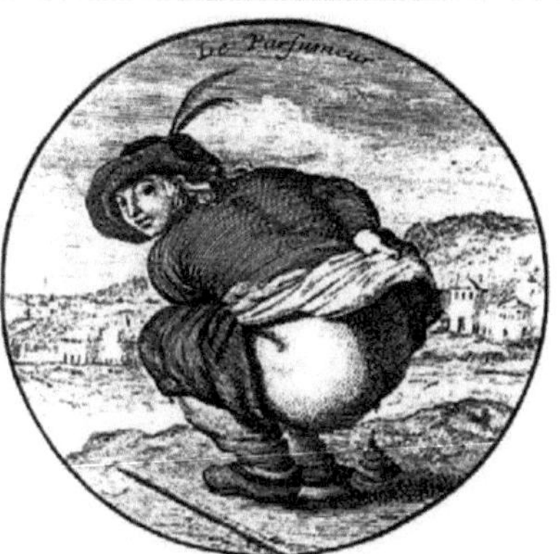

16th century drawing of a person defecating in squatting position outside

The defecation cycle

In the adult human, the process of defecation, or the defecation cycle, is normally a combination of both voluntary and involuntary processes. The defecation cycle is the interval of time between the completion of one defecation, and the completion of the following defecation. At the start of the cycle, the rectal ampulla (anatomically also: *ampulla recti*) acts as a temporary storage facility for the unneeded material. As additional fecal material enters the rectum, the rectal walls expand. A sufficient increase in fecal material in the rectum causes stretch receptors from the nervous system located in the rectal walls to trigger the contraction of rectal muscles, relaxation of the internal anal sphincter and an initial contraction of the skeletal muscle of the external sphincter. The relaxation of the internal anal sphincter causes a signal to be sent to the brain indicating an urge to defecate.

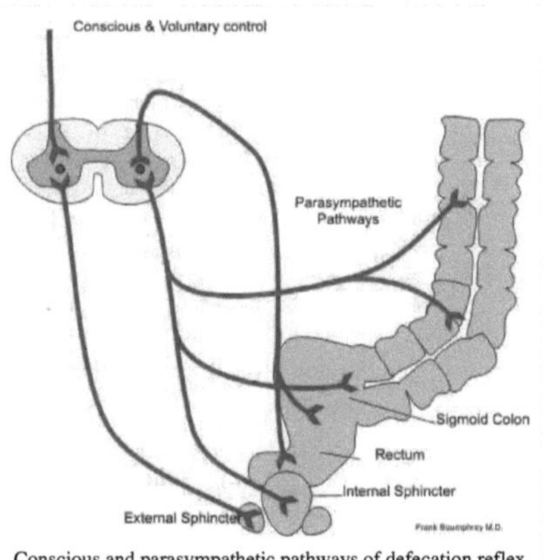

Conscious and parasympathetic pathways of defecation reflex

If this urge is not acted upon, the material in the rectum is often returned to the colon by reverse peristalsis where more water is absorbed, thus temporarily reducing pressure and stretching within the rectum. The additional fecal material is stored in the colon until the next mass 'peristaltic' movement of the transverse and descending colon. If defecation is delayed for a prolonged period the fecal matter may harden and autolyze, resulting in constipation.

Once the voluntary signal to defecate is sent back from the brain, the final phase of the cycle begins. The rectum now contracts and shortens in peristaltic waves, thus forcing fecal material out of the rectum and out through the anal canal. The internal and external anal sphincters along with the puborectalis muscle allow the feces to be passed by pulling the anus up over the exiting feces in shortening and contracting actions.

Muscular aspects

Defecation is normally assisted by taking a deep breath and trying to expel this air against a closed glottis (Valsalva maneuver). This contraction of expiratory chest muscles, diaphragm, abdominal wall muscles, and pelvic diaphragm exert pressure on the digestive tract.

Cardiovascular aspects

During defecation, the thoracic blood pressure rises,[1] and as a reflex response the amount of blood pumped by the heart decreases. Death has been known to occur in cases where defecation causes the blood pressure to rise enough to cause the rupture of an aneurysm or to dislodge blood clots (see thrombosis). Also, in terminating the Valsalva maneuver, blood pressure falls; this, often coupled with standing up quickly to leave the toilet, results in a common incidence of fainting.

Neurological aspects

When defecating, the external sphincter muscles relax. The anal and urethal sphincter muscles are closely linked, and experiments by Dr. Harrison Weed at the Ohio State University Medical Center have shown that they can be contracted only together, not individually, and that they both show relaxation during urination. This explains why defecation is frequently accompanied by urination, and why urination is frequently accompanied by flatulence.

Defecation may be involuntary or under voluntary control. Young children learn voluntary control through the process of toilet training. Once this has been achieved, loss of control causing fecal incontinence may be caused by physical injury – such as damage to the anal sphincter that may result from an episiotomy, intense fright, excessive pressure placed upon the abdomen, inflammatory bowel disease, impaired water absorption in the colon (diarrhea), and psychological or neurological factors.

The loss of voluntary control of defecation is experienced frequently by those undergoing a terminal illness.[2]

Posture aspects

The positions and modalities of defecation are culture-dependent. The natural and instinctive method used by all primates, including humans for defecation, is the squatting position.[3] Squat toilets, sometimes referred to as 'natural-position toilets', are still used by the vast majority of the world, including most of Africa and Asia. The widespread use of seated-position toilets in the Western World is a recent development, beginning in the 19th century with the advent of indoor plumbing.[4]

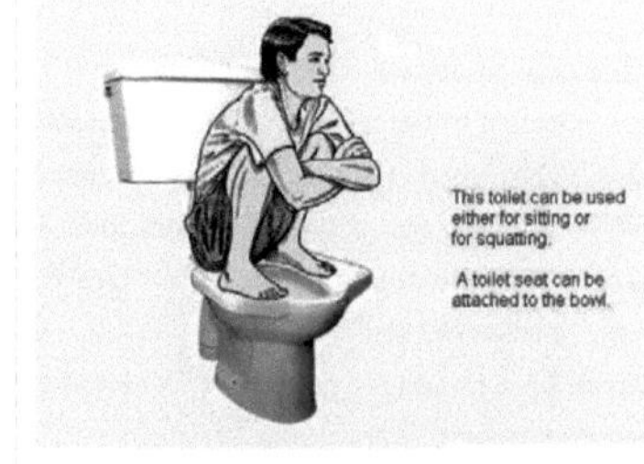

This toilet can be used
either for sitting or
for squatting.
A toilet seat can be
attached to the bowl.
Defecation in squatting position

Bockus in *Gastroenterology*, the standard textbook on the subject, states:

> The ideal posture for defecation is the squatting position, with the thighs flexed upon the abdomen. In this way the capacity of the abdominal cavity is greatly diminished and intra-abdominal pressure increased, thus encouraging expulsion ...[5]

Cleaning

The anus and buttocks may be cleansed with toilet paper, similar paper products, or other absorbent material. In some cultures water is used (e.g. as with a bidet or lota) either in addition or exclusively. In Japan and South Korea, some toilets known as washlets are designed to wash and dry the anus of the user after defecation.

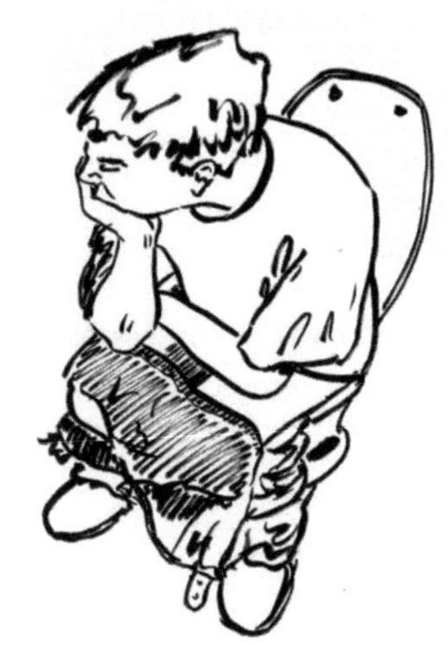

Defecation in sitting position

See also

- Coprophilia
- Laxative

References

Notes

[1] Defecation (http://www.britannica.com/EBchecked/topic/155613/defecation), Encyclopedia Britannica

[2] Joanne Lynn, MD. Merck. October 2007. Symptoms During a Fatal Illness (http://www.merck.com/mmhe/sec01/ch008/ch008f.html). Uploaded 3/1/09.

[3] Kira A. The Bathroom. Harmondsworth: Penguin, 1976, revised edition, pp.115,116.

[4] A History of Technology, Vol.IV: The Industrial Revolution, 1750-1850. (C. Singer, E Holmyard, A Hall, T. Williams eds) Oxford Clarendon Press, pps. 507-508, 1958

[5] Bockus. Gastroenterology. p. 754 2nd ed. Saunders, Philadelphia and London, 1964

Bibliography

- Widmaier, Raff, Strang (2006). "Vanders Human Physiology, the mechanisms of body function. Chapter 15. McGraw Hill.

Human physiology

Human physiology is the science of the mechanical, physical, bioelectrical, and biochemical functions of humans in good health, their organs, and the cells of which they are composed. In simple terms "Human Physiology" is the study of the body and its functions in each of the different system in any living body .Physiology focuses principally at the level of organs and systems. Most aspects of human physiology are closely homologous to corresponding aspects of animal physiology, and animal experimentation has provided much of the foundation of physiological knowledge. Anatomy and physiology are closely related fields of study: anatomy, the study of form, and physiology, the study of function, are intrinsically tied and are studied in tandem as part of a medical curriculum.

The concept of homeostasis

The term "Homeostasis" refers to the maintenance of overall inner resistance in the body. Homeostatic stable the body by regulating internal environment at the body surface.These kinds of conditions are requited in order to make body keep functioning. Homeostatic procedure is essential for the survival of each cell.Homeostasis in a general sense refers to stability, balance or equilibrium. Maintaining a stable internal environment requires constant monitoring and adjustments as conditions change. This adjusting of physiological systems within the body is called homeostatic regulation.

Systems

Traditionally, the academic discipline of physiology views the body as a collection of interacting systems, each with its own combination of functions and purposes.Each body system contributes to the homeostasis of other systems and of the entire organism. No system of the body works in isolation, and the well-being of the person depends upon the well-being of all the interacting body systems.

	System	Clinical study	Physiology
	The **nervous system** consists of the central nervous system (which is the brain and spinal cord) and peripheral nervous system. The brain is the organ of thought, emotion, and sensory processing, and serves many aspects of communication and control of various other systems and functions. The **special senses** consist of vision, hearing, taste, and smell. The eyes, ears, tongue, and nose gather information about the body's environment.	neuroscience, neurology (disease), psychiatry (behavioral), ophthalmology (vision), otolaryngology (hearing, taste, smell)	neurophysiology
	The **musculoskeletal system** consists of the human skeleton (which includes bones, ligaments, tendons, and cartilage) and attached muscles. It gives the body basic structure and the ability for movement. In addition to their structural role, the larger bones in the body contain bone marrow, the site of production of blood cells. Also, all bones are major storage sites for calcium and phosphate.	osteology (skeleton), orthopedics (bone disorders)	cell physiology, musculoskeletal physiology
	The **circulatory system** consists of the heart and blood vessels (arteries, veins, capillaries). The heart propels the circulation of the blood, which serves as a "transportation system" to transfer oxygen, fuel, nutrients, waste products, immune cells, and signalling molecules (i.e., hormones) from one part of the body to another. The **blood** consists of fluid that carries cells in the circulation, including some that move from tissue to blood vessels and back, as well as the spleen and bone marrow.	cardiology (heart), hematology (blood)	cardiovascular physiology
	The **respiratory system** consists of the nose, nasopharynx, trachea, and lungs. It brings oxygen from the air and excretes carbon dioxide and water back into the air.	pulmonology.	respiratory physiology

	The **gastrointestinal system** consists of the mouth, esophagus, stomach, gut (small and large intestines), and rectum, as well as the liver, pancreas, gallbladder, and salivary glands. It converts food into small, nutritional, non-toxic molecules for distribution by the circulation to all tissues of the body, and excretes the unused residue.	gastroenterology	gastrointestinal physiology
	The **integumentary system** consists of the covering of the body (the skin), including hair and nails as well as other functionally important structures such as the sweat glands and sebaceous glands. The skin provides containment, structure, and protection for other organs, but it also serves as a major sensory interface with the outside world.	dermatology	cell physiology, skin physiology
	The **urinary system** consists of the kidneys, ureters, bladder, and urethra. It removes water from the blood to produce urine, which carries a variety of waste molecules and excess ions and water out of the body.	nephrology (function), urology (structural disease)	renal physiology
	The **reproductive system** consists of the gonads and the internal and external sex organs. The reproductive system produces gametes in each sex, a mechanism for their combination, and a nurturing environment for the first 9 months of development of the offspring.	gynecology (women), andrology (men), sexology (behavioral aspects) embryology (developmental aspects)	reproductive physiology
	The **immune system** consists of the white blood cells, the thymus, lymph nodes and lymph channels, which are also part of the lymphatic system. The immune system provides a mechanism for the body to distinguish its own cells and tissues from alien cells and substances and to neutralize or destroy the latter by using specialized proteins such as antibodies, cytokines, and toll-like receptors, among many others.	immunology	immunology
	The **endocrine system** consists of the principal endocrine glands: the pituitary, thyroid, adrenals, pancreas, parathyroids, and gonads, but nearly all organs and tissues produce specific endocrine hormones as well. The endocrine hormones serve as signals from one body system to another regarding an enormous array of conditions, and resulting in variety of changes of function.	endocrinology	endocrinology

The traditional divisions by system are somewhat arbitrary. Many body parts participate in more than one system, and systems might be organized by function, by embryological origin, or other categorizations. In particular, is the "**neuroendocrine system**", the complex interactions of the neurological and endocrinological systems which together regulate physiology. Furthermore, many aspects of physiology are not as easily included in the traditional organ system categories.

The study of how physiology is altered in disease is pathophysiology.

Feedback system

The reaction of body from the changes of the internal and external environment called " Feedback System".There are mainly two types of the Feedback system 1)Negative Feedback system 2)Positive Feedback system.Negative feedback: a reaction in which the system responds in such a way as to reverse the direction of change. Since this tends to keep things constant, it allows the maintenance of homeostasis.Positive feedback: a response is to amplify the change in the variable. This has a destabilizing effect, so does not result in homeostasis. Positive feedback is less common in naturally occurring systems than negative feedback, but it has its applications. [1]

See also

- Comparative physiology
- Darwinian medicine
- Evolutionary psychology
- Krogh Principle
- Physiology
- Thrifty phenotype

References

[1] "HUMAN PHYSIOLOGY" (http://upload.wikimedia.org/wikimedia/en-labs/c/cd/Human_Physiology.pdf). Wikibooks. . Retrieved 17 December 2011.

Further reading

- Babsky, Evgeni; Boris Khodorov, Grigory Kositsky, Anatoly Zubkov (1989). Evgeni Babsky. ed. *Human Physiology, in 2 vols.*. Translated by Ludmila Aksenova; translation edited by H. C. Creighton (M.A., Oxon). Moscow: Mir Publishers. ISBN 5-03-000776-8.
- Sherwood, Lauralee (2010) (Hardcover). *Human Physiology from cells to systems* (7 ed.). Pacific Grove, CA: Brooks/cole. ISBN 978-0495391845.
- Provophys (C) Whiteknight (C) RiRi82 (C) Jcran69 (C) Scout21972 (C) · Jtervortn (C) · DorothyD (C) · VWilkes (C) · Jacquel (C) · Danyellmarie (C) · Keith davis (C) · Mperkins (C) · Never2late (C) · Shellybird2 (C) · BriannaLenford (C) · Jen A (C) · Pwoodson (C) · Nataliehaveron (C) · Melissasmith (C) · Brentwaldrop (C) (2006-2007). "1" (http://upload.wikimedia.org/wikimedia/en-labs/c/cd/Human_Physiology.pdf) (Ebook). Wikibooks contributors. pp. 1–10.

Notes

External links

- Human Physiology textbook at Wikibooks

Enteroendocrine cell

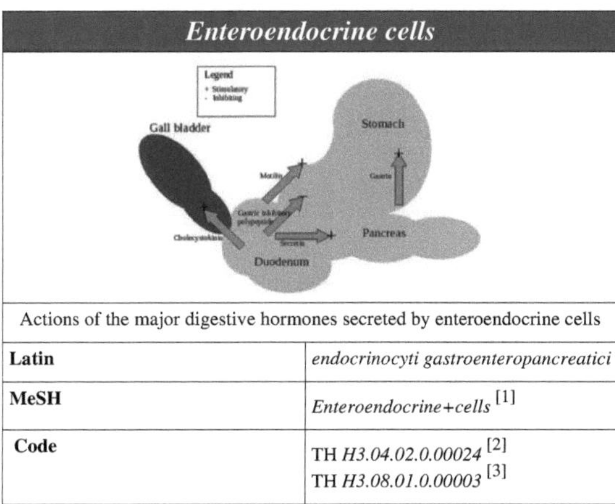

Actions of the major digestive hormones secreted by enteroendocrine cells

Latin	*endocrinocyti gastroenteropancreatici*
MeSH	*Enteroendocrine+cells* [1]
Code	TH *H3.04.02.0.00024* [2] TH *H3.08.01.0.00003* [3]

Enteroendocrine cells are specialized endocrine cells of the gastrointestinal tract. They produce hormones such as serotonin[4] , somatostatin, motilin, cholecystokinin, gastric inhibitory peptide, neurotensin, vasoactive intestinal peptide, and enteroglucagon.

Most enteroendocrine cells are found in the islets of Langerhans, but they are also found in other locations. For example, the G cells (which secrete gastrin) are located primarily in the stomach.[5] Enteroendocrine cells are also found in the duodenum.[6]

Enterochromaffin-like cell and enterochromaffin cells are also considered enteroendocrine cells.[7]

Pathology

Rare and slow growing carcinoid tumors develop from these cells. When a tumor arises it has the capacity to secrete large volumes of hormones.

See also

- APUD cell

References

[1] http://www.nlm.nih.gov/cgi/mesh/2011/MB_cgi?mode=&term=Enteroendocrine+cells
[2] http://www.unifr.ch/ifaa/Public/EntryPage/ViewTH/THh304.html
[3] http://www.unifr.ch/ifaa/Public/EntryPage/ViewTH/THh308.html
[4] UIUC Histology Subject *321* (https://histo.life.illinois.edu/histo/atlas/oimages.php?oid=321)
[5] *iv_1/g/G_cell* (http://www.medcyclopaedia.com/library/topics/volume_iv_1/g/G_cell.aspx) article at GE's Medcyclopaedia
[6] Histology at BU *11604loa* (http://www.bu.edu/histology/p/11604loa.htm) - "Endocrine System: duodenum, enteroendocrine cells"
[7] MeSH *Enteroendocrine+cells* (http://www.nlm.nih.gov/cgi/mesh/2011/MB_cgi?mode=&term=Enteroendocrine+cells)

Enterochromaffin cell

Enterochromaffin cell	
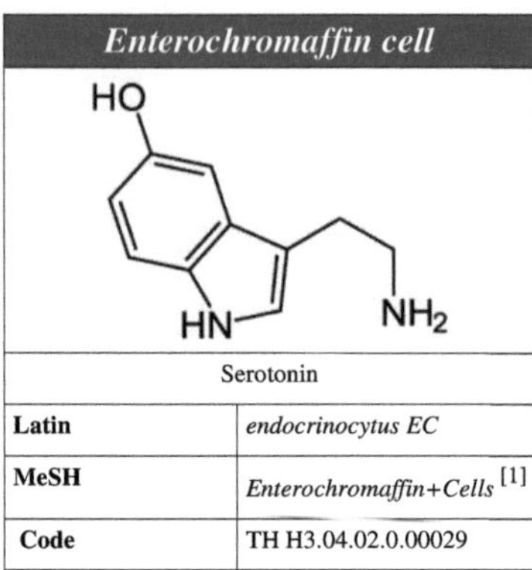	
Serotonin	
Latin	*endocrinocytus EC*
MeSH	*Enterochromaffin+Cells* [1]
Code	TH H3.04.02.0.00029

Enterochromaffin (EC) cells (**Kulchitsky cells**) are a type of enteroendocrine cell[2] occurring in the epithelia lining the lumen of the digestive tract and the respiratory tract.

Function

They contain about 90% of the body's store of serotonin (5-HT).[3]

In the gastrointestinal tract, 5-HT is important in response to chemical, mechanical or pathological stimuli in the lumen. It activates both secretory and peristaltic reflexes, and activates vagal afferents (via 5-HT_3 receptors) that signal to the brain (important in the generation of nausea). Ondansetron is an antagonist of the 5-HT_3 receptor and is an effective anti-emetic.

They are stimulated by gastrin, a molecule that is produced at the antrum of the stomach by G cells.

Origin

They are derived from neural crest.[4]

The enterochromaffin cells are derived from the same stem cells as the rest of the epithelium, and are not derived from the migratory neural crest source that provides the enteric nervous system. [5]

Etymology

They are called "entero"[6] meaning related to the gut and "chromaffin" because of a chromium salt reaction that they share with chromaffin cells of the adrenal medulla (adrenal glands). [7]

"Enterochromaffin-like cells"

Another population of chromaffin cells is found only in the stomach wall, called enterochromaffin-like cells (ECL). They look like EC cells but do not contain 5-HT.

ECL cells respond to gastrin released by G-cells and they release histamine, which will stimulate the parietal cells to produce gastric acid.

Pathophysiology

Neuroendocrine progenitor cells in the bronchial epithelium, the progenitors to Kulchitsky cells, have been implicated in the origin of small cell lung cancer. [8]

See also

- Carcinoid syndrome
- Serotonin

References

[1] http://www.nlm.nih.gov/cgi/mesh/2011/MB_cgi?mode=&term=Enterochromaffin+Cells

[2] MeSH *Enterochromaffin+Cells* (http://www.nlm.nih.gov/cgi/mesh/2011/MB_cgi?mode=&term=Enterochromaffin+Cells)

[3] Josef Donnerer; Fred Lembeck (2006). *The chemical languages of the nervous system: history of scientists and substances* (http://books.google.com/books?id=HkOhFssK5UIC&pg=PT161). Karger Publishers. pp. 161–. ISBN 9783805580045. . Retrieved 23 May 2011.

[4] Tao Le; Vikas Bhushan; Neil Vasan (1 January 2010). *First Aid for the USMLE Step 1, 2010* (http://books.google.com/books?id=eVAtPktgw0UC&pg=PA119). McGraw Hill Professional. pp. 119–. ISBN 9780071633406. . Retrieved 11 November 2010.

[5] Thompson M, Fleming KA, Evans DJ, Fundele R, Surani MA, Wright NA (October 1990). "Gastric endocrine cells share a clonal origin with other gut cell lineages". *Development* **110** (2): 477–81. PMID 2133551.

[6] Entero- definition - Medical Dictionary definitions of popular medical terms easily defined on MedTerms (http://www.medterms.com/script/main/art.asp?articlekey=3258)

[7] *1516961798* (http://www.gpnotebook.co.uk/simplepage.cfm?ID=1516961798) at GPnotebook

[8] eMedicine - Lung Cancer, Small Cell : Article by Abid Irshad (http://www.emedicine.com/radio/topic405.htm)

APUD cell

APUD cells constitute a group of apparently unrelated endocrine cells, which were named by the scientist A.G.E. Pearse, who developed the APUD concept in the early 60's. These cells share the common function of secreting a low molecular weight polypeptide hormone. There are several different types which secrete the hormones secretin, cholecystokinin and several others. The name is derived from an acronym, referring to the following:[1] [2]

Actions of the major digestive hormones secreted by APUD cells

- **A**mine - for high amine content.
- **P**recursor **U**ptake - for high uptake of (amine) precursors.
- **D**ecarboxylase - for high content of the enzyme amino acid decarboxylase (for conversion of precursors to amines).

See also

- Apudoma
- Enteroendocrine cell
- Neuroendocrine cell

References

[1] Welbourn RB (January 1977). "Current status of the apudomas". *Ann. Surg.* **185** (1): 1–12. doi:10.1097/00000658-197701000-00001. PMC 1396259. PMID 12724.

[2] Pearse, A.G. (1969). "The cytochemistry and ultrastructure of polypeptide hormone-producing cells of the APUD series and the embryologic, physiologic and pathologic implications of the concept". *J. Histochem. Cytochem.* **17** (5): 303–13. PMID 4143745.

External links

- *-328531944* (http://www.gpnotebook.co.uk/simplepage.cfm?ID=-328531944) at GPnotebook
- MeSH *APUD+Cells* (http://www.nlm.nih.gov/cgi/mesh/2011/MB_cgi?mode=&term=APUD+Cells)

Article Sources and Contributors

Segmentation contractions *Source*: http://en.wikipedia.org/w/index.php?title=Segmentation_contractions *Contributors*: Arcadian, Bwpach, DarkFalls, Delldot, 4 anonymous edits

Esophagus *Source*: http://en.wikipedia.org/w/index.php?title=Esophagus *Contributors*: 3strang3d, A More Perfect Onion, Aatxox, Abcdefg 12345, Absconded Northerner, Abstraktn, Academic Challenger, Acdx, Agateller, Ageekgal, Ahoerstemeier, Akanemoto, Alansohn, Alex.tan, Alfie66, Alpine88, Amhurley, Anatomist90, Anaxial, Anclation, Andres, Angusmclellan, Anna Frodesiak, Antandrus, Arcadian, Arjun024, Arthena, AtTheCoast, AxelBoldt, Azquelt, Badgernet, Basharh, Beansmeanshines, Bencherlite, Betacommand, BiT, Binary TSO, Bockbockchicken, Boing! said Zebedee, Bomac, Brichcja, Brittany.benda, BryanG, Btyner, CAD6DEE2E8DAD95A, Clreland, Capricorn42, Carlo.milanesi, Caval valor, Cburnett, Christian List, Ckatz, Countryfan276, Creation7689, Cwds, Czechrite, DARTH SIDIOUS 2, DVD R W, Daven200520, Dcfleck, Delldot, Diberri, Dictabeard, Dina, DoctorC, DogcatcherDrew, Doktory, DoubleBlue, Dpeters11, Dr.cardwell, Drgarden, E2eamon, Eleassar, Epbr123, Faetie, Falcon8765, Feministo, Finngall, Flyguy649, Foobaz, Fred Ratcliff, Freecat, Fæ, Gadfium, Geoffrey, GetAgrippa, Glacialfox, Grafen, Gravecat, Grover cleveland, Gulmammad, Haham hanuka, Hakufu Sonsaku, Harps21, Hfwd, Hordaland, Horologium, Hu12, Hveziris, Hydrogen Iodide, Imnotminkus, J.delanoy, JVinocur, Ja 62, Jaknouse, Jaranda, Jesse Viviano, Jmeeter, Jmundo, Jni, Johnelson, Jose77, Jpogi, Julesd, Juliancolton, Jusjih, KaiserPeter, Kaobear, Kcordina, Kingpin13, KlingonDoctor, Kmoor92, Knucmo2, Knutux, KoshVorlon, Kostisl, Kristof vt, LAX, Lambiam, Laurap414, Lcarsdata, LeilaniLad, Lisatwo, Logan, Lucas.Josef, Luka Krstulović, Lupin, Mac, Marek69, MarkS, Maxim, Mephistophelian, Michael Hardy, Mikael Häggström, Mike2vil, Mikemoral, Milton.mic, Mithaca, Mud, N5iln, NHRHS2010, Natalie Erin, NawlinWiki, Nephron, Netha Hussain, NewEnglandYankee, Nikopoley, Nilepierre, Nistra, Njufas, Nlu, Noctibus, Nonexistant User, Nunh-huh, Nxl256, Nytimes19992000, Pandaman13, Paranomia, Paxsimius, Pedro, PeteThePill, Philip Trueman, Pit, Primaler, Professsor, Quakemistress, Quartertone, Quartonoffolis, Qwyrxian, R9tgokunks, Ragumani, Raysonho, Recognizance, Renato Caniatti, RichardF, Richardcavell, Ronz, SMcCandlish, Samir, SeaValeYen, Sesu Prime, Shawndkc, Sheeana, Sir Stig, Sirmelle, SkyWalker, Sligocki, Slodave, Spartan, Sprachmeister, Staticshakedown, Stemonitis, StephP, Stevenfruitsmaak, StradivariusTV, TaintedMustard, Tarquin, Tbackstr, Teemu Maki, Template namespace initialisation script, The Thing That Should Not Be, TheOtherJesse, TheProject, TheTrojanHought, Theseven7, Three-quarter-ten, Tide rolls, Tofugod10, Tohd8BohaithuGh1, Torrente, Tweedledee123, Udo.schroeter, UkPaolo, Unschool, Utcursch, Vary, Versus22, ViolinGirl, Vishnava, Vladaig, Vogon77, Void main, Vrenator, Vörös, Waycool27, WelshMatt, Whitecloth, Why Not A Duck, Whysofxckingserious, Wiensgov, WikipedianMarlith, Wikipelli, Yidisheryid, Yodoekeyo, Zundark, Zyqqh, 522 anonymous edits

Peristalsis *Source*: http://en.wikipedia.org/w/index.php?title=Peristalsis *Contributors*: 10014derek, Achill, Adrian, AlistairMcMillan, AlvinPing, Amire80, Andrea105, Arc de Ciel, Arcadian, ArmadilloFromHell, Armoreno10, Aua, BLACKMONGOOSE13, Biomenne, Bluemoose, Boing! said Zebedee, BrianKnez, Brighterorange, Bryan Derksen, Cbritt4, Chinju, Chrisjj, Chumpster9, Cmcnicoll, Cool3, Curb Chain, Cybercobra, DarkArcher, Delldot, DerHexer, Discosammich, Dogposter, Dougofborg, Drmies, Echuck215, Elnerdo, Emw, Engr Shaukat ALI, Epbr123, Esrob, FF2010, Fennec, Grayshi, HCA, Hob Gadling, InvictaHOG, J.delanoy, Jahiegel, Janetyler, Jfurr1981, Jimmy Hammerfist, Jmundo, John254, Judicatus, Kinema, Knowledgeum, KongminRegent, Kpjas, Logan, Malcolm Morley, Manufracture, Mario1952, Materialscientist, Matt Deres, Meewam, Metju, Michaelandtpain, Mike.lifeguard, Miniyazz, Mixs, Neutrality, Nubiatech, Oidhche, Palica, PierreAbbat, Pinethicket, Praefectorian, Randwicked, RickK, Robertaedwards, Ronhjones, Samwb123, Sceptre, Shanoman, Shunju-kun, Someone else, SpaceFlight89, Spitfire, Strabismus, Sundar, Tabercil, Tb, Temporaluser, The Drizzlemeister, The Utahraptor, Therearewaytoomanybooksinhere, Tide rolls, Van der Hoorn, Velella, WLU, Wikielwikingo, Wimt, Winchelsea, Wlodzimierz, Wtmitchell, Xasxas256, Zambani, 250 anonymous edits

Small intestine *Source*: http://en.wikipedia.org/w/index.php?title=Small_intestine *Contributors*: A. B., ABF, Abeg92, Ablonus, Achurch, Acullum, Aitias, Akanemoto, Aksi great, Alansohn, Aldis90, Alex.tan, Allen4names, Alpha Quadrant (alt), Altimmons, Anatomist90, Anaxial, Andrew73, Anetode, Antandrus, Arcadian, Archer3, ArglebargleIV, Armando Navarro, AsphyXy, Auxiliary Watchlist, Avb, Avnjay, Avoided, Basharh, Beaumont, Beyond silence, Bhadani, BiT, Blanchardb, Bluemoose, Bobo192, Bomac, BrokenSegue, Bryan986, Budgy Speedwagon, Can't sleep, clown will eat me, CapitalR, Capricorn42, Captain panda, Captinhippie, Cburnett, Celticsrule, Chaojoker, Ched Davis, Chloeobrian, Chris G, Christian75, Cntras, Cometstyles, Conserrnd, D, DDima, Dalziel 86, DanielCD, Darth Mike, Dave6, Davewild, Davis Capella, Dclayh, Decltype, Delldot, DerHexer, Devourer09, Dingar, Docboat, Dolive21, Drgarden, Elmaynardo, Elmer Clark, Epbr123, Ericdn, Everyking, Excirial, FF2010, Facts707, Fan Railer, Farside6, Fdp, Fieldday-sunday, Flyguy649, Foxtrotman, Fredwerner, Freecat, Freezing the mainstream, Freiza2k1, Frymaster, Fuzzbucket123, GHe, Gastro-en, Ghaleonh41, Giftlite, Ginsengbomb, Glacious, GlassCobra, Glimz, Gogo Dodo, Grafen, Graham87, Gregp99, Gscshoyru, Gz33, H665555336666, Haham hanuka, Headd, Heron, Hfwd, Hi i like chocolate, Hotshot977, Hrodulf, Hut 8.5, Ice Cold Beer, Idcmp, Igksb, InfoCan, Insanity Incarnate, InverseHypercube, Iridescent, Irishguy, IronGargoyle, Isnow, Ixfd64, J.delanoy, JForget, JR98664, Ja 62, Jackfork, Jacoplane, Janon2, Jaredpickles, Jfdwolff, Jhenderson777, JinJian, Jobnikon, Joelmills, Jordan Yang, Jsbf, Julesd, Ka34, Kazvorpal, Keegan, Keilana, Khukri, Kingpin13, Kiswanson, Kityates, Knutux, Kpjas, Kseym3, Kubigula, Kudret abi, LFaraone, Latics, LearnAnatomy, Lectonar, Leolaursen, Les boys, Lesotho, Levil, Light current, Lipothymia, Lisap, Lmcelhiney, Longy77, Lupo, MER-C, MONGO, Mac, Mahela007, Mardochaios, MarkMarek, Martinl, Master2841, Math Champion, Mayooranathan, Merovingian, Metsavend, MightyWarrior, Mikael Häggström, Mike Christie, Miquonranger03, Mishuletz, Moe Epsilon, Mortense, Mpereza, Mr genius94, MrArifnajafov, MrEskimo0, Muad, Mygerardromance, NHRHS2010, Natgoo, NatureA16, NawlinWiki, Nelly4, Nephron, NerdyScienceDude, NeuroE, NewEnglandYankee, Ngantengyuen, Nick2crosby, Nina Gerlach, Norm, Nsaa, Nv8200p, Obradovic Goran, OlEnglish, Ombudsman, Ouishoebean, OwenX, Paul August, Pdcook, PeregrineV, Pharaoh of the Wizards, Philip Trueman, Pi, Pinethicket, PoccilScript, Pol430, Prashanthns, Premeditated Chaos, Professor marginalia, Pruitlgoe, Psy guy, Puchiko, Puhlaa, Pwhitwor, Qxz, R'n'B, RA0808, Ranveig, Ratznium, Razimantv, Razorflame, Reinyday, Renwick, Rettetast, RexNL, Rgoodermote, Rhopkins8, Rjanag, Rjwilmsi, Roberta F., Rodri316, Ronhjones, Samir, Samrolken, SchfiftyThree, Scientizzle, Seaphoto, Sethpt, Shadowjams, Shellac, Shenme, Shlomke, Shoshonna, Shrumster, Sien324, Simonfairfax, SlightlyMad, Sluzzelin, Smappy, Smirkster, Some jerk on the Internet, Soph121, Stan Shebs, StaticGull, Stubblyhead, Suitequal, SuperHamster, Swid, Syrthiss, TangLab, Tasc, Taurusrat, Tazaliiscool, Techman224, TehBrandon, Teletubbie26, Template namespace initialisation script, Tgeairn, The Anome, The Thing That Should Not Be, TheMightyOrb, TheTrojanHought, Theda, Thingg, Tide rolls, Tiggerjay, Timir2, Tohd8BohaithuGh1, Tomdo08, Ucanlookitup, Uirauna, Underjack, Uniquely Fabricated, Unschool, Vanished user 39948282, Vera.tetrix, Voyagerfan5761, Vrenator, Vshehu, WatermelonPotion, Wayne Slam, West.andrew.g, Wikineopet, WikipedianMarlith, Wikipelli, Willtron, Wilsonjd, Wisnuops, Wknight94, WojPob, Wouterstomp, WriterHound, Ww, Xhaoz, Xitit, Yamamoto Ichiro, Yekrats, Yngvadottir, Ysabellaflemflem, Zenazn, Zsinj, Zumlin, Zzuuzz, 885 anonymous edits

Large intestine *Source*: http://en.wikipedia.org/w/index.php?title=Large_intestine *Contributors*: -), 1roo13, 2D, 2help, ABF, Abbieboitz, Addshore, Akanemoto, Alansohn, Allen4names, Allens, Ame09, American Eagle, Anaxial, Andres, Angusmclellan, Appleboy, Arakunem, Arcadian, Arthena, Ascidian, Avoided, BCube, Basharh, Beyond silence, Boivie, Bongwarrior, Boulaur, BrokenSegue, Bubble13 94, C messier, Caerwine, Cammydizzle, Can't sleep, clown will eat me, Capricorn42, Captain-n00dle, Carmichael95, Cedders, Chaojoker, Chris G, Chuckiesdad, Chun-hian, Ckatz, Connormah, Conortodd, Cowardly Lion, Ctjf83, Cxz111, Cyfal, DO11.10, Daflasha, Dancingteen, DarkFalls, Davidruben, Deadlytrian, Decltype, Deli nk, Delldot, Discospinster, Docu, DoubleBlue, Drphilharmonic, E2e3v6, Edward321, Elisabeth33, Eliz81, Emma202, Epbr123, Eptin, Fabioli2010, Facts707, Favonian, Felix1101, Felyza, Fergking, Fiberglass Monkey, Fire Effects, FreddyKrueger69, Freecat, Fuzheado, Gene93k, Ghislain Montvernay, Gilliam, Glacialfox, Glacious, GlobeGores, Gloopty, Grafen, Graham87, GrayFullbuster, Hariva, Harold f, Helios87, Hobartimus, Huffameg, Husond, Ijustam, Iketsi, Inferno, Lord of Penguins, Iridos, Ixfd64, J. Spencer, J.delanoy, Jackfork, Jaimie Henry, JamesBWatson, Javawizard, Javert, Jevansen, JinJian, JohnCD, Jojit fb, Jovianeye, Jrkonen, Juliancolton, Justintime516, KJS77, KTo288, Kanonkas, Keilana, Khalid Mahmood, KirbyRandolf, Kittiekatsu, Kizor, Koyos, L Kensington, LOL, LaMenta3, Lam Kin Keung, LeaveSleaves, LedgendGamer, Leeearnest, Legolost, Llywelyn2000, Lukep913, Lyellin, M8trix228, Macy, MakOwak0, Marcus Brute, Marek69, MarsRover, Massimo Macconi, MasterXC, Maurice Termeer, MaxSem, Maxipuchi, Maxxicum, Mayooranathan, Meekywiki, Meldor, Methecooldude, Metsavend, Michaelas10, Micki, Mikael Häggström, Mindstalk, Minorthoughts, Moipaulochon, Mortense, MosheA, Mrut1780, Nagy, NawlinWiki, Neargonad, NerdyScienceDude, NewEnglandYankee, Ngantengyuen, Nick Number, Nickr95, Nivix, Nk, Non-dropframe, Nono64, Northumbrian, Nurg, Onorem, Orchew, Ouishoebean, Pewwer42, Philip Trueman, PierreAbbat, Piperh, Plainpaper, Polapopsd, Portalmaster50, PrincessofLlyr, Pro crast in a tor, Puffin, Pyrrhus16, Quantumobserver, RA0808, Ranveig, Reaper Eternal, Reaperman, Red Winged Duck, Regardless143, Renamed user 1407, Rettetast, RexNL, Rich Farmbrough, Roberta F., Rokyfox, SETh of MONROVIA, Sanawon, Santista1982, SchfiftyThree, Science4sail, Sean D Martin, Sean Heron, Sharks1249, Shirulashem, Sirmelle, Skela, Slakr, Slon02, Snowolf, SoLando, Soliloquial, SpaceFlight89, Spartan-James, Spitfire, Squids and Chips, SteinbDJ, Stevertigo, Storm Rider, Suitequal, Sundar, Sutjo-18005, THEN WHO WAS PHONE?, Tanzania, TenOfAllTrades, The Thing That Should Not Be, TheEgyptian, TheMightyOrb, Tide rolls, Timir2, Tins128, Tocant, Tom Lougheed, Toys72196, TrekCaptainUSA, Triona, Trusilver, TucsonDavid, Uberpotato, Uhai, Unschool, Vanished User 1007, Vanished user 39948282, Vidariv, Virtig01, WLU, Wendell, Wiensgov, WikipedianMarlith, Wikipelli, WilliamKF, Willtron, Willyv1, Wjejskenewr, Yamamoto Ichiro, Yerpo, Yock1, Yomangani, Yosri, Zaparojdik, ןדָ ןושארו, احمد.غامدي.24, 548 anonymous edits

Gastrointestinal physiology *Source*: http://en.wikipedia.org/w/index.php?title=Gastrointestinal_physiology *Contributors*: Amalas, Animeronin, Arcadian, Beeswaxcandle, Caerwine, Cdt129, Connaboi, Davidarpeters, Devourer09, Finlay McWalter, Gobonobo, Nick Number, Rjwilmsi, Ronz, VAcharon, 19 anonymous edits

Digestion *Source*: http://en.wikipedia.org/w/index.php?title=Digestion *Contributors*: 07sutherlanda, 28421u2232nfenfcenc, ABF, Abb615, Abfackeln, Abrech, Acroterion, AeoniosHaplo, Ahoerstemeier, Aida CZ, Alansohn, Ale jrb, Alexbrewer, Alexius08, AlexiusHoratius, Alfonzo Smarty, Alpha 4615, Alphachimp, Alqari, Altzinn, Amberrock, Amog, Andrev, Andreworkney, Andrewrp, Andy85719, Anghrist, Angusmclellan, Annypants, Anthemos, Anthonyhcole, Antonio Lopez, Arakunem, Arcadian, Arcanedude91, Architect76, Arjun01, Art LaPella, Arthena, Arvind0602, Ashok1, Asikhi, Atlant, AtomicDragon, AuburnPilot, Aydinapkar16, Bachrach44, Banalnatae, Banes, Batsnumbereleven, Beano, Beland, Ben Ben, Ben parr2004, Benbread, BendersGame, Bennylin, BertieB, Betterusername, Bgd135guy, Bijou39, Billyg, Bkkbrad, Bkonrad, Blabberfruit, Blahblah670, Bobandjerry, Bobo192, Bobthebuilder11, BoganBoy, Bogey97, Boing! said Zebedee, Bomac, Bongwarrior, BorgHunter, Boulaur, Brazul2, BrianGV, Brody014, Bronsonboy, Brougham96, Bsadowski1, Bucephalus, Burn874, C'est moi, CPColin, Cactus.man, Cacycle, Cacycle test, Caknuck, Caltas, Camw, Can't sleep, clown will eat me, Canis Lupus, CanisRufus, Capitalistroadster, Capricorn42, Captain-tucker, CardinalDan, Carlosguitar, Casablanca2000in, CaseyPenk, Catdoctor, Catgut, Celarnor, Centuriono, Chamal N, Chamberlian, Chanleesheng, Chaojoker, ChaoticGhost, Ched Davis, Cheetolayne15, Chickenfajitas, Chillirocks!!!, Christian75, Christinexuelian, Chuunen Baka, Ckatz, Clicketyclack, Closedmouth, Clutch7337, Compellingelegance, Cooper091496, Corinne68, Corpx, Correct24, Cpillay2, Cst17, Csurprise, D sam charles, D. Recorder, DARTH SIDIOUS 2, DVD Smith, Darkdadaah, Darkfight, David Eppstein, David spector, Davidovic, Davidr222, Dbfirs, Deagle AP, Decltype, Delldot, Denisarona, Diannaa, Diberri, DickFagit, Diogeneselcinico42, Discospinster, Diz syd 63, Dlohcierekim's sock, Dmitri Yuriev, Dmohan12345, Donarreiskoffer, DoubleBlue, Doulos Christos, Drilnoth, Drmies, DubaiTerminator, Duncan, Dwhutton, Dwmr, Dycedarg, E2e3v6, Ebraminio, Ecogreg2009, EconoPhysicist, Eddturtle, Edgar181, Edison, Edward, Edward321,

Elenseel, Elipongo, Eliz81, Ember of Light, EmmaPJs, Enuja, Enviroboy, Epbr123, Eras-mus, Eric-Wester, Erik9, Esrob, Euchiasmus, Ewen, Ewlyahoocom, Excirial, Falcon4fly, Falcon8765, Faradayplank, Farosdaughter, Fieldday-sunday, Fir0002, Fireice, Fish 13579, Fisher99wat3, Flewis, Fluffernutter, FlyHigh, Fountain Lake, Frankeinstein, Frankenpuppy, Fruchogurt, Fuzheado, Fæ, GB fan, GT5162, GanLnkZld, Gcpeoples, Geekdiva, Geeteshgadkari, Geneb1955, Geoff Wing, Ggghhhkkk, Gilliam, Ginsengbomb, Giraffedata, Glane23, Glass Sword, GlassCobra, Golbez, Goldkingtut5, Grafen, Graft, Greensburger, Grim23, Gunnar SJ, Gurchzilla, Guycalledryan, Hadal, Hard Sin, Hargo kapay, Hydriz, Hydrogen Iodide, Hópur 5, I platypus, II MusLiM HyBRiD II, IRP, Ianbu, Ibbn, Iceman1337, Imjustmatthew, Immunize, ImperatorExercitus, ImperfectlyInformed, Iridescent, Irishman0477, IronGargoyle, Isnow, Itfc+canes=me, Ixfd64, J.delanoy, J04n, JForget, JR98664, Jack Schlederer, Jackelfive, Jackol, Jacob.jose, Jakkeven, Jaknouse, JamesAM, Jamesontai, Jan eissfeldt, Jauhienij, JavierMC, Javierito92, JayC, Jeepday, Jengod, Jfdwolff, Jhenderson777, Jiddisch, Jim1138, Jimothytrotter, JinJian, Jmundo, Jncraton, Joanjoc, Jobe layton, Joehall45, JohnFromPinckney, Jojhutton, Jojit fb, Jomunro, Jondel, Joodeak, Jovianeye, Jpeeling, JubalHarshaw, Julesd, Juliaschopick, Junglecat, Jusdafax, Jwpurple, KGasso, Karenjc, Katalaveno, Keelm, Kemiv, Kevin42, Khalid Mahmood, Khukri, Killiondude, Kingpin13, Kissekatt, Kjkolb, KnowledgeBased, KnowledgeOfSelf, Kobinks, Kongu1, Kpjas, Krich, Kubigula, KungFuRealTalk, L Kensington, LFaraone, La Pianista, LalalaSausageMoo, LedgendGamer, Ledmonkey, Leeannedy, Leroylevine, Liddleheart, Life, Liberty, Property, Lights, Lilsteven589, Lir, Lisatwo, Lithpiperpilot, Liulab, LizardJr8, Lovenoble, LovesMacs, Lradrama, Lukeduke5, Luna Santin, Lupo, MER-C, Mac, MadeBlindxxx, Malcolmxl5, Mandarax, Manlyman123, Marauder40, Marek69, Marshallsumter, Mashaunix, Materialscientist, Mato, Matt Deres, Matthew Yeager, Mattisse, Max Naylor, Mbuddemeyer, McSly, Meaghan, Mechwarrior Puppies, Mendors, Mentifisto, Mgiganteus1, Microtony, Mikael Häggström, Mikaey, Mike6271, Millahnna, Mindboom, Minderbinder, Misibacsi, Mmkemikal, Modulatum, Monoshiri, Morning277, Moverton, Mr. Lefty, Mrzaius, Mspraveen, Munita Prasad, Mursaleen Ahmad, Mutinus, N419BH, NPTV, Naddy, Nathan, NathanoNL, Naturalmetal, NawlinWiki, Necromancer44, Neptunefire, NewEnglandYankee, Nicolae Coman, Nk, Nneonneo, NocturnalHorde, Noformation, Notreallydavid, Nsaa, Nuttycoconut, Nymphetaminechild, Onceonthisisland, Oore, Osm agha, Otolemur crassicaudatus, Ouishoebean, OverlordQ, Oxymoron83, PCHS-NJROTC, PFHLai, PaterMcFly, Patriarch, Paul August, Paul Slocum, Pdcook, Pearle, Pedrora, Persian Poet Gal, Phantomsteve, Pharaoh of the Wizards, Phatom87, Philip Trueman, Phoebe, Piano non troppo, Pinethicket, Pingveno, PirateMonkey, Pishaww, Pit, Pitom112397, PlaysWithLife, Pmsyyz, PoccilScript, Polly, Popenfresh123, Possum, Pradeep93, PranksterTurtle, Pred, Pro crast in a tor, Pro-Lick, Prunesqualer, Qpcstom, R R Carney, R'n'B, RAWR54321, Rama4, Randall Nortman, Ranveig, Rck314, Reach Out to the Truth, Readopedia, Reaper Eternal, Reconsider the static, RedRollerskate, Redskinsrock23, Reihaneh, Renato Caniatti, Renzo joongeun, Res2216firestar, Rettetast, RexNL, Riana, Rich Farmbrough, Richard New Forest, Rickspawn96, Riffraffselbow, Rishi.bedi, Rituraj110, Rjwilmsi, Robert Bond, Rofl, Roger Roger, Ronhjones, Ronz, Rothefyre, RoyBoy, Rrburke, Rror, Ruby.red.roses, Rumiton, Runningonbrains, Ruyter, Ryoutou, SJP, Sakkura, Salt Worm, Samuel phd, Sandgem Addict, Sbowers3, SchfiftyThree, Seahorseruler, Seb az86556, Sephiroth BCR, Sheldony120, Shentino, Shirina, Shlomke, Sidhekin, Simon12, Sir1, SirLeopold, Sirprojects, Sixbluemooses, Sjakkalle, Sjb90, Sjö, Skittleys, Skunkboy74, Slon02, Slowking Man, Smartdogz123456, Smartse, Smeira, Snowolf, Spaceman85, SpearowMAX, Speedevil, Staffwaterboy, Star27, Stealth500, Steel, Stellaxio, Stephenb, Strait, Strombollii, Suffusion of Yellow, SunCreator, TaintedCherub, Tandle134, Taylornate, Tedder, Tekks, Tellyaddict, Tempodivalse, Thaistory, The High Fin Sperm Whale, The Rambling Man, The Random Editor, The Thing That Should Not Be, The Utahraptor, The stuart, TheTito, Thedjatclubrock, Thingg, Tide rolls, Tiptoety, Tohd8BohaithuGh1, Tom.k, TonyClarke, Tonyng84, Torswin, TreadingWater, Tregoweth, Treisijs, Tresiden, Trevor MacInnis, Truebluepassword, Tryptofish, Tydude187, UISKuwait, Ulric1313, Ultimate77, Umeshghosh, Uncle Dick, Undoubtedly0, Usb10, Useight, User A1, User27091, VMS Mosaic, Vaux, Versus22, Vinceouca, Vipinhari, Voltron, Vortexrealm, VoxLuna, Vssun, WLU, Waggers, WatermelonPotion, Wavehunter, Wavelength, Wayne Slam, Westonomor181, Westoonomor181, Wiensgov, WikHead, Wiki alf, WikiLaurent, Wikiblythe, Wikidsoup, Wikidudeman, Wikimichael22, WikipedianMarlith, Wikipelli, Willtron, Wimt, Wimvandorst, Wknight94, Wuhwuzdat, Ww, Wyatt915, XSxDxRx, Xx mwa, XxCRYxx095, Yekrats, Yerpo, YouareAguy, Ysheng, Yukiesue, ZB8640, Zaharous, Zakhalesh, Zaphod Beeblebrox, Zephalis, Zhou Yu, Ziggurat, Zodiac2415, Zodon, ÌnfoCan, ملاني, 1930 anonymous edits

Migrating motor complex *Source*: http://en.wikipedia.org/w/index.php?title=Migrating_motor_complex *Contributors*: Arcadian, Cmcnicoll, Creidieki, Gastro-en, InvictaHOG, OlEnglish, The Land, Timothydavie, 9 anonymous edits

Borborygmus *Source*: http://en.wikipedia.org/w/index.php?title=Borborygmus *Contributors*: AdeMiami, Airmint1, Alan Liefting, Alex.tan, Altenmann, Arcadian, Augen Zu, Baastuul, BarryTheUnicorn, Benpage26, Biomenne, Bryan Derksen, Butsuri, Calaka, Cchhrriiss, Cholga, Cmcnicoll, Davidbspalding, DeutscherStahl, Doremo, Fredrik, Gobonobo, GrFTER, Graham87, Imrankhan85, Jackbanana, Jfdwolff, JohnJSal, JohnnyRuin, Juliancolton, Kellychoi, Kevspencer, Kuru, Kwamikagami, LER223, Luna Santin, Lycanthrope777, Meco, Metropolitan90, Mhbourne, Michael A. White, MikeCooper15, Millahnna, Offalian, Oldman, PBP, Paxsimius, Pekinensis, Phthinosuchusisanancestor, Piksi, Pixor, PloniAlmoni, Quandaryus, R'n'B, Retodon8, Reza luke, Ringbang, Rockfang, Rsabbatini, Thorns among our leaves, Vitriden, Yobmod, דוד55, 62 anonymous edits

Defecation *Source*: http://en.wikipedia.org/w/index.php?title=Defecation *Contributors*: (aeropagitica), -), -Frank-, .mdk., 041744, 1silver11, 21655, 24fan24, 6'5Guy, 64jesse4567, ABF, AGK, AbJ32, Adashiel, Addshore, AdeMiami, Afctenfour, Ageekgal, Agüeybaná, Ahoerstemeier, Ahriik, Aircorn, Aisere, Aitias, Aka042, Akamad, Alansohn, Ale jrb, Alex.tan, Alexius08, Ali K, Altenmann, Ameliorate!, Ammubhave, Andreas Erick, Andrewbonnell, AndrewvdBK, Andy M. Wang, Angusr95, Anilocra, Animum, Anna Lincoln, Anonymous Dissident, Appleberry33, Apurv1980, Arcadian, Armeria, Arthena, Ash, AshleyX3, Ashanda, Astroview120mm, Atleastimnotfat1, Atulrules, Avono, Avraham, Avrilfan2604, Ayla, BMXxRASTAbanana, Ballhairkillaz, Balmer21210, Barrelroll20, Bassman5, Beasthero, Beaub95, Beccabombom, Beckettc, Becky Sayles, Beebeegurl11, Beeswaxcandle, Before My Ken, Bento00, Betacommand, Beyond My Ken, Bforte, Bgedwards, Bigfan213, Bills16309, Bjarki S, Bkkbrad, BlazeTheMovieFan, Blehfu, Blow of Light, Bluerasberry, Bobo192, Bongwarrior, Boredgurl182, Brampel121, Brandon, Brian Crawford, Brianga, Brion VIBBER, Brossow, BryanGx, Bubuka, Buchanan-Hermit, Bumble123, Byeitical, C5221, CBDunkerson, COA320, Caj123123123, Calvin 1998, Camsynth, Can't sleep, clown will eat me, CanadianLinuxUser, Canterbury Tail, CapitalR, CardinalDan, Catgut, CatherineMunro, Causa sui, Cflm001, Chaldean, CharlotteWebb, Cheeseniblets69, Chitomcgee, Chris the speller, Chris9086, Chriswaterguy, CiTrusD, Cincle, Circeus, Cjsmed, Clemwang, Click23, CoNaDa, Codycody2062, Cometstyles, CommonsDelinker, Conti, Cosmic Latte, Cosmic.space.turtle, Courcelles, Cpl Syx, Craig Pemberton, Crazycomputers, Cremepuff222, Crithit5000, CuttableName, D, D6, DARTH SIDIOUS 2, Dabomb87, Damicatz, Daniel Olsen, DannyKitty, Dark Lord of the Sith, Darkspots, David.Monniaux, DavidJ710, Dawnseeker2000, DaydreamBeliever1, Dbach, Ddllsas, DeadEyeArrow, Deathawk, Decoy, Defunctzombie, Delldot, Demonslave, Dennis Brown, DerHexer, Deryck Chan, Devon1, Devrit, Diannaa, Dicknyabooty, Diety, Dillard421, Dina, Dinkytown, Discospinster, Djheini, Docboat, Doddy Wuid, Doompiggy, DoubleJJ, DougsTech, Doulos Christos, Dpr, Dreadstar, DreamHaze, Dukeofwulf, DurinsBane87, Dycedarg, ENpeeOHvee, Earlypsychosis, EdGl, Eduardo Sellan III, Eeekster, Efglol, Elcobbola, Elipongo, Elsenrail, EncMstr, Enti342, EoGuy, Epbr123, EronMain, Erunestian, Euryalus, Eveninja, Evil Monkey, Excirial, Eyeon, Fangbao de Van, Fartsaton, Fatfart555, Ferenj, Fieldday-sunday, Finalius, Fire emblem 4127, Fireinacrowdedtheatre, FiveRings, Fivexthethird, Flarn2006, Flashbrah, Floppy Face, Frankypwns, Freekee, Freshacconci, Funeral, Furrykef, Fyyer, Fæ, GEARY4, GEORGEalso, GTZ-44-ecosan, Gabidibella, Gabwej, Gaming3ever, Gary13579, Gdo01, Genya Avocado, George100, Ghostfacearchivist, Ghosts&empties, Gigemag76, Gilliam, Gjask, Glacialfox, Gogo Dodo, Golbez, Goodvac, GorillaWarfare, Gotbass7, GraemeL, Grafen, Grreat56, Grundle2600, Gsp8181, Gtstricky, Gurch, Hacker1012929348, Hadal, Hajatvrc, HalJor, Halfgiant9000's awesome pet, Hamdevguru, Hamtechperson, Hans Adler, Hariva, Henrik, Heron, Heshyjesse, Hirishaan, Hirohisat, Hixface, Hollywood6258, Hookman07, Horia96, Horseperson12345, Humanbeing123456, Husnock, Hut 6.5, Hydrogen Iodide, I dream of horses, IRP, IW.HG, Iamjameson, Icairns, IceUnshattered, Idontknow123441a, Imme1020, Iridescent, Ishanz, Itgeek2002, Ixfd64, J. Spencer, J.delanoy, JKaver018, JaGa, Jacek Kendysz, Jackfork, Jackol, Jake4423678, Jared Preston, JasonHockeyGuy, Javlin munky, Jdforrester, Jesse Mills, Jfdwolff, Jimgawn, Jlitton12, JoanneB, JodyB, JodyBayne, John254, Jojhutton, Jonathan108, Jonathan2400, Josh3580, Joshua Scott, Jpark3909, Jpgordon, Julesd, Juliancolton, Jusdafax, Justforasecond, Kablammo, Kapowaz, Kaptainlauren, Karafias, Katalaveno, Kbh3rd, Keilana, Kencurran, Keserman, Kickmeitalk1, Kieran544, Killiondude, Kingpoobah, Kinkyturnip, Kminnis, KnowledgeOfSelf, Koavf, Krymson, Kubigula, Kungfuadam, Kungming2, Kuru, Kyle Barbour, LCVVandal, LaMenta3, Ladys man5000, Landon1980, LarryHouse54, Lars Washington, Latka, Law, LeaveSleaves, LedgendGamer, Lessthanthree, Lfitzge1, LibLord, Ling.Nut, Lipothymia, Liu Bei, Lloydpick, Logan, Logologist, LonelyMarble, Lucepapoose, Ludicrousfeline, Luna Santin, MBisanz, MER-C, MacGyverMagic, Maddie omg, Madhero88, MageStealth, Magioladitis, Mahewa, Majorly, Malinaccier, Man of destiny, Maniac18, Manure, Marauder40, Margaritaville2009, Martin451, Mas 18 dl, Maskedbas tard, Mattar123, Maxwell Derwinee, MaxxFordham, McSly, Mcbill88, Mcflie, Meaghan, Meeples, Mentifisto, MercyMine, Merlinsorca, Mikael Häggström, Mike Payne, Mike Rosoft, Mild Bill Hiccup, Miles, Minghong, Minna Sora no Shita, Miquonranger03, MisterSanderson, Modemac, Monkey Bounce, Monkeycheez, Montgomery '39, MosheA, MrWhich, Muchosucko, Musical Linguist, Musiphil, Mwanner, MyLogicIsUndenyable, Mysteriousman132, N5iln, Nagy, Nancy, Narom, NawlinWiki, NeilN, NerdyNSK, Nickptar, Nido, Nightman81, Nightscream, Nihiltres, Nn123645, Noah Salzman, Nohat, Noobeditor, NotAnonymous0, Notgood, Nsnlover112233, Nurg, OHWiki, Oda Mari, Ohnoitsjamie, OlEnglish, Oliver202, Ollie the Magic Skater, Olly150, Omicronpersei8, Oneiros, Onorem, Orange Suede Sofa, Otolemur crassicaudatus, Ouada'Ruhn, OwenX, Oxymoron83, PDH, PSYCHO, Palica, Panoptical, Panser Born, Paramorelove43, Passargea, Patiwat, Patrick, Paul August, Paulbalegend, Paulinho28, Pcarter7, Penbat, Persian Poet Gal, Peruvianllama, Peter Chastain, Peter Karlsen, PeterSymonds, Philip Trueman, PhilxCrAzY, Phpscriptcoder, Piano non troppo, Pichpich, PierreAbbat, Pigeonattak, Pill, Pineapple breath, Pingveno, Pinkadelica, Pixie3243, Ploppies, Pmanc, Poop4705, Poop4873258, Porqin, Prashanthns, President Rhapsody, Proofreader77, Pseudomonas, Pu35yl1cker11, Punkedagain, Purpleroxy1019, Pwninator5000, Pxma, Qleem, Quintote, Quirk, Qwfp, R'n'B, RA0808, RadLink5, RadioActive, Radon210, Rahulk2.0, RainbowOfLight, Ral315, RandomAct, RandomStringOfCharacters, Raven in Orbit, RayAYang, Razorflame, Rbarreira, Rdsmith4, Rdw uiuc, Reconsider the static, Res2216firestar, RexNL, Rhi151223, Rhobite, Richard n, Richard001, Richi, Rlmaorr, Robert185, Robinlobb, Robomaeyhem, Robrox0009, Rockstar imn, Ronhjones, Rory096, Rotlagler wackoman, Rrburke, Rsscp1, Rubberduckies, Rukario639, Ryan R0olz, Rybo1993, SJP, SKANKYAGUILERA, SWAdair, SWFan00, Saayiit, Sagsaw, Sampi, Sanbeg, Sandwich Eater, Satori Son, Saturn star, SchfiftyThree, Scottperry, Scotty vela, Scwlong, Seaphoto, Secret22314, Shadowjams, Shawn in Montreal, Shipwreck jim, Shirulashem, Shoeofdeath, Sivret20, Sjö, Sk8n4life1212, Skarebo, Skiryder4life, Skizzik, Sky Attacker, Solidmantis, Sometimesthinking, SpaceFlight89, Specs112, Spitfire19, Spoom, Springeragh, Stephenb, Steven Zhang, Subino, Suffusion of Yellow, SupaStarGirl, Super travis, SuperHamster, Supra guy, Susfele, SweetNeo85, Sxim3xi, THEN WHO WAS PHONE?, Tamajared, Tapir Terrific, Tbhotch, Techman224, Tedius Zanarukando, Teles, TenOfAllTrades, Tenjikuronin, The Rambling Man, The Thing That Should Not Be, The way, the truth, and the light, TheGerm, Thecheesykid, Theda, Theleftorium, Thenderson, Theroguex, Thescrambles1, Thingg, Thue, Thumbee, Tiddly Tom, Tide rolls, TigerShark, Tim1357, TimBentley, Tinton5, Tinytime, Tlim7882, Tobyc75, Tom harrison, Tommy2010, Tony Fox, Toon05, TrashMan10, Trey, Trigaranus, Triona, Tristanb, Trusilver, Tslocum, Turtles111, TutterMouse, Ugen64, Ukexpat, Ukimono101, Uncle Dick, Unyoyega, Urmomish, Uthbrian, Vanished user 39948282, Vcelloho, Verbal, Versageek, Versus22, Viele&sons, Vipinhari, Virus326, WCWBF, WadeSimMiser, WaiHing, Wenli, Weyes, WhisperToMe, Wi-king, Wiki alf, WikiKatie4, Wikipoints4wiki, Wikipooper123, Willking1979, Wing zero 100, Wizardman123, Wknight94, Woohookitty, Work permit, Worldedixor, Wwbamfdo, Wysprgr2005, X!, XxxASLxxx, Y0ugotn03rd, Yourname, Zachlipton, Zanimum, Zbaseball16, Zh, Zigger, Zisimos, Zzuuzz, Île flottante, 1214 anonymous edits

Human physiology *Source*: http://en.wikipedia.org/w/index.php?title=Human_physiology *Contributors*: AED, Addingrefs, Altenmann, Alteripse, Amikake3, Andrewrp, Animeronin, Apostrophyx, Arcadian, B, Barneca, Barticus88, Beelaj., Bensaccount, Born2flie, BoundaryRider, CALR, Celeritas, CommonsDelinker, Corpx, Cureden, Cuthbertwong, DabMachine, Diberri, DivineAlpha, Doctorthigpen, El C, Eliz81, Epbr123, Erud, Euryalus, Evolauxia, Excirial, Fp26-NJITWILL, Fran Rogers, Fribbler, Galoubet, Giftlite, Glstar6, Gregogil, Harry, JForget, JR98664, JamesBWatson, Jfdwolff, Jnyanydts, Johnny C. Morse, Knowledge Seeker, Koavf, La Pianista, LeCire, Leon..., LikeHolyWater, Lillianremus, LittleHow, MK8, Manticore, Maurreen, Mayumashu, Mentifisto, Mr.Bip, Mugregg, Nafile, Nehrams2020, NeoChaosX, Ngb, Nihiltres, Nithinchand, Nono64, Opelio, Parhamr, Pax:Vobiscum, Pbroks13, PeaceNT, Petiatil, PhatRita,

PoccilScript, Provophys, R'n'B, Res2216firestar, RexNL, Rich Farmbrough, SCEhardt, Shoeofdeath, Solus ipse Inc., Stepa, Szquirrel, Tazmaniacs, Tcncv, Teles, TenOfAllTrades, Tide rolls, TimBentley, Timichal, Tommy2010, Uthbrian, Veron, Vsmith, Vuong Ngan Ha, W.stanovsky, Wapondaponda, WereSpielChequers, Whatamldoing, Whatiguana, Whoelius, Wikinonymous, Wouterstomp, Zotel, 109 anonymous edits

Enteroendocrine cell *Source*: http://en.wikipedia.org/w/index.php?title=Enteroendocrine_cell *Contributors*: Arcadian, Caerwine, Critical Info, Eikenhein, Leolaursen, Nee622, Nephron, O keyes, Shokod, Tekks, 3 anonymous edits

Enterochromaffin cell *Source*: http://en.wikipedia.org/w/index.php?title=Enterochromaffin_cell *Contributors*: Arcadian, Benlavan, ChrisCork, CopperKettle, Daedalus-Prime, Diberri, Finlay McWalter, Gigemag76, Hodja Nasreddin, Imnotminkus, It Is Me Here, Koene, MedicShaft, Paulpb, Peco15, Rjjaramillo, Rjwilmsi, Serephine, V8rik, Wisdom89, Woohookitty, 28 anonymous edits

APUD cell *Source*: http://en.wikipedia.org/w/index.php?title=APUD_cell *Contributors*: Arcadian, Beeswaxcandle, Chaoborus, CopperKettle, Deviator13, IceCreamAntisocial, Nephron, Oldgreeneyes, RDBrown, Rjwilmsi, Rubiweiss, Tekks, 4 anonymous edits

Image Sources, Licenses and Contributors

Image:Illu01 head neck.jpg *Source*: http://en.wikipedia.org/w/index.php?title=File:Illu01_head_neck.jpg *License*: unknown *Contributors*: User:Arcadian

Image:BauchOrgane wn.png *Source*: http://en.wikipedia.org/w/index.php?title=File:BauchOrgane_wn.png *License*: unknown *Contributors*: + my_update

File:Relations of the aorta, trachea, esophagus and other heart structures.png *Source*: http://en.wikipedia.org/w/index.php?title=File:Relations_of_the_aorta,_trachea,_esophagus_and_other_heart_structures.png *License*: unknown *Contributors*: User:Mikael Häggström, User:ZooFari

File:Thorax section 2.jpg *Source*: http://en.wikipedia.org/w/index.php?title=File:Thorax_section_2.jpg *License*: unknown *Contributors*: User:Anatomist90

File:Tinción hematoxilina-eosina.jpg *Source*: http://en.wikipedia.org/w/index.php?title=File:Tinción_hematoxilina-eosina.jpg *License*: unknown *Contributors*: w:en:User:SamirSamir@enwiki

File:Illu esophageal layers.jpg *Source*: http://en.wikipedia.org/w/index.php?title=File:Illu_esophageal_layers.jpg *License*: unknown *Contributors*: Arcadian, Origamiemensch, 1 anonymous edits

File:Mid_esophageal_mass.jpg *Source*: http://en.wikipedia.org/w/index.php?title=File:Mid_esophageal_mass.jpg *License*: unknown *Contributors*: Original uploader was Samir at en.wikipedia

File:Illu stomach2.jpg *Source*: http://en.wikipedia.org/w/index.php?title=File:Illu_stomach2.jpg *License*: unknown *Contributors*: Arcadian, High Contrast, Jacklee, Origamiemensch, Rory096

File:Digestive system showing bile duct.png *Source*: http://en.wikipedia.org/w/index.php?title=File:Digestive_system_showing_bile_duct.png *License*: unknown *Contributors*: AKA MBG, Bemoeial2, Frieda, 4 anonymous edits

File:Illu dige tract.jpg *Source*: http://en.wikipedia.org/w/index.php?title=File:Illu_dige_tract.jpg *License*: unknown *Contributors*: Arcadian, Bobarino, MichaelFrey

File:Illu esophagus.jpg *Source*: http://en.wikipedia.org/w/index.php?title=File:Illu_esophagus.jpg *License*: unknown *Contributors*: training.seer.cancer.gov

File:Gray384.png *Source*: http://en.wikipedia.org/w/index.php?title=File:Gray384.png *License*: unknown *Contributors*: Arcadian

File:Gray503.png *Source*: http://en.wikipedia.org/w/index.php?title=File:Gray503.png *License*: unknown *Contributors*: Arcadian

File:Gray994.png *Source*: http://en.wikipedia.org/w/index.php?title=File:Gray994.png *License*: unknown *Contributors*: Arcadian, Bemoeial2, Hellerhoff, Magnus Manske, Tarawneh, Was a bee

File:Gray1032.png *Source*: http://en.wikipedia.org/w/index.php?title=File:Gray1032.png *License*: unknown *Contributors*: Arcadian, Magnus Manske

File:Gray1033.png *Source*: http://en.wikipedia.org/w/index.php?title=File:Gray1033.png *License*: unknown *Contributors*: Arcadian, Magnus Manske, Origamiemensch

File:Gastro-esophageal jxn.JPG *Source*: http://en.wikipedia.org/w/index.php?title=File:Gastro-esophageal_jxn.JPG *License*: unknown *Contributors*: Jpogi

File:Herpes esophagitis - high mag.jpg *Source*: http://en.wikipedia.org/w/index.php?title=File:Herpes_esophagitis_-_high_mag.jpg *License*: unknown *Contributors*: User:Nephron

File:Esophagus 1.jpg *Source*: http://en.wikipedia.org/w/index.php?title=File:Esophagus_1.jpg *License*: unknown *Contributors*: User:Anatomist90

Image:Peristaltic.jpg *Source*: http://en.wikipedia.org/w/index.php?title=File:Peristaltic.jpg *License*: unknown *Contributors*: Biomenne

Image:Peristalsis.gif *Source*: http://en.wikipedia.org/w/index.php?title=File:Peristalsis.gif *License*: unknown *Contributors*: User:Auawise

Image:Earthworm movement all.jpg *Source*: http://en.wikipedia.org/w/index.php?title=File:Earthworm_movement_all.jpg *License*: unknown *Contributors*: Mokele at en.wikipedia

Image:Stomach_colon_rectum_diagram.svg *Source*: http://en.wikipedia.org/w/index.php?title=File:Stomach_colon_rectum_diagram.svg *License*: unknown *Contributors*: Indolences created it on the English Wikipedia.

File:Small intestine.jpg *Source*: http://en.wikipedia.org/w/index.php?title=File:Small_intestine.jpg *License*: unknown *Contributors*: User:Anatomist90

Image:Small intestine low mag.jpg *Source*: http://en.wikipedia.org/w/index.php?title=File:Small_intestine_low_mag.jpg *License*: unknown *Contributors*: User:Nephron

Image:Gray849.png *Source*: http://en.wikipedia.org/w/index.php?title=File:Gray849.png *License*: unknown *Contributors*: Arcadian, Magnus Manske

Image:Gray1224.png *Source*: http://en.wikipedia.org/w/index.php?title=File:Gray1224.png *License*: unknown *Contributors*: Arcadian, Quibik, 1 anonymous edits

Image:Intestine-diagram.svg *Source*: http://en.wikipedia.org/w/index.php?title=File:Intestine-diagram.svg *License*: unknown *Contributors*: User:Connormah

Image:Gray1223.png *Source*: http://en.wikipedia.org/w/index.php?title=File:Gray1223.png *License*: unknown *Contributors*: Arcadian, Bryan, Bukk, Gyógymasszőr Békáson, Jacklee, 3 anonymous edits

Image:Digestive system diagram en.svg *Source*: http://en.wikipedia.org/w/index.php?title=File:Digestive_system_diagram_en.svg *License*: unknown *Contributors*: User:LadyofHats

image:Bacterial Conjugation en.png *Source*: http://en.wikipedia.org/w/index.php?title=File:Bacterial_Conjugation_en.png *License*: unknown *Contributors*: Mike Jones

Image:VFT ne1.JPG *Source*: http://en.wikipedia.org/w/index.php?title=File:VFT_ne1.JPG *License*: unknown *Contributors*: Aroche, BRUTE, ComputerHotline, Denis Barthel, NoahElhardt, 2 anonymous edits

Image:Trophozoites of Entamoeba histolytica with ingested erythrocytes.JPG *Source*: http://en.wikipedia.org/w/index.php?title=File:Trophozoites_of_Entamoeba_histolytica_with_ingested_erythrocytes.JPG *License*: unknown *Contributors*: Der Lange, Patho, Wlodzimierz

Image:Ara hybrid - Catalina Macaw.jpg *Source*: http://en.wikipedia.org/w/index.php?title=File:Ara_hybrid_-_Catalina_Macaw.jpg *License*: unknown *Contributors*: Original uploader was Skyler13 at en.wikipedia

Image:Squid beak measuring.jpg *Source*: http://en.wikipedia.org/w/index.php?title=File:Squid_beak_measuring.jpg *License*: unknown *Contributors*: Linél, Mgiganteus

Image:Carcharodon megalodon P1060082.jpg *Source*: http://en.wikipedia.org/w/index.php?title=File:Carcharodon_megalodon_P1060082.jpg *License*: unknown *Contributors*: User:Amphibol

Image:Abomasum (PSF).png *Source*: http://en.wikipedia.org/w/index.php?title=File:Abomasum_(PSF).png *License*: unknown *Contributors*: Airelle, Bob Burkhardt, Jak, Kersti Nebelsiek

File:Flesh fly concentrating food.jpg *Source*: http://en.wikipedia.org/w/index.php?title=File:Flesh_fly_concentrating_food.jpg *License*: unknown *Contributors*: User:Fir0002

Image:Digestive system diagram edit.svg *Source*: http://en.wikipedia.org/w/index.php?title=File:Digestive_system_diagram_edit.svg *License*: unknown *Contributors*: User:Alvesgaspar, User:LadyofHats

image:Digestive hormones.jpg *Source*: http://en.wikipedia.org/w/index.php?title=File:Digestive_hormones.jpg *License*: unknown *Contributors*: Tekks (talk). Original uploader was Tekks at en.wikipedia

Image:Bernard Picart - The Perfumer.jpg *Source*: http://en.wikipedia.org/w/index.php?title=File:Bernard_Picart_-_The_Perfumer.jpg *License*: unknown *Contributors*: Bernard Picart

File:Defecation reflex.png *Source*: http://en.wikipedia.org/w/index.php?title=File:Defecation_reflex.png *License*: unknown *Contributors*: User:Boumphreyfr

Image:Pedestal-squat-toilet.jpg *Source*: http://en.wikipedia.org/w/index.php?title=File:Pedestal-squat-toilet.jpg *License*: unknown *Contributors*: User:Jonathan108

Image:Defecation img 1907.jpg *Source*: http://en.wikipedia.org/w/index.php?title=File:Defecation_img_1907.jpg *License*: unknown *Contributors*: User:Rama

Image:Human brain NIH.jpg *Source*: http://en.wikipedia.org/w/index.php?title=File:Human_brain_NIH.jpg *License*: unknown *Contributors*: OldakQuill, StuRat, Talgraf777, Ysangkok, 1 anonymous edits

Image:Skelett-Mensch-drawing.jpg *Source*: http://en.wikipedia.org/w/index.php?title=File:Skelett-Mensch-drawing.jpg *License*: unknown *Contributors*: Er Komandante, Hellerhoff, Jodo, Origamiemensch, Petwoe, Snek01, 1 anonymous edits

Image:Diagram of the human heart (cropped).svg *Source*: http://en.wikipedia.org/w/index.php?title=File:Diagram_of_the_human_heart_(cropped).svg *License*: unknown *Contributors*: User:Yaddah

Image:heart-and-lungs.jpg *Source*: http://en.wikipedia.org/w/index.php?title=File:Heart-and-lungs.jpg *License*: unknown *Contributors*: Gray's Anatomy

Image:Stomach colon rectum diagram.svg *Source*: http://en.wikipedia.org/w/index.php?title=File:Stomach_colon_rectum_diagram.svg *License*: unknown *Contributors*: Indolences created it on the English Wikipedia.

Image:Skin-no language.PNG *Source*: http://en.wikipedia.org/w/index.php?title=File:Skin-no_language.PNG *License*: unknown *Contributors*: Coyau, Leridant

Image:Gray1120.png *Source*: http://en.wikipedia.org/w/index.php?title=File:Gray1120.png *License*: unknown *Contributors*: Aktron, Diberri, GeorgHH, German, Lennert B, Maksim, Roxbury-de, SterkeBak, 1 anonymous edits

Image:Male anatomy.png *Source*: http://en.wikipedia.org/w/index.php?title=File:Male_anatomy.png *License*: unknown *Contributors*: Ephraim33, Frank C. Müller, Lennert B, Odedee, Ranveig, Saperaud, Stephanie, Tsaitgaist, Xiong Chiamiov

Image:PBNeutrophil.jpg *Source*: http://en.wikipedia.org/w/index.php?title=File:PBNeutrophil.jpg *License*: unknown *Contributors*: Dirk Hünniger, Lennert B, Santosga, 1 anonymous edits

Image:Illu endocrine system.png *Source*: http://en.wikipedia.org/w/index.php?title=File:Illu_endocrine_system.png *License*: unknown *Contributors*: Alfie66, Ankarali99, Dany 123, Giowilrogubar, Intermedichbo, Istvánka, Lennert B, Manuelt15, Metju, Origamiemensch, Was a bee, 18 anonymous edits

Image:Digestive hormones.jpg *Source*: http://en.wikipedia.org/w/index.php?title=File:Digestive_hormones.jpg *License*: unknown *Contributors*: Tekks (talk). Original uploader was Tekks at en.wikipedia

Image:Serotonin (5-HT).svg *Source*: http://en.wikipedia.org/w/index.php?title=File:Serotonin_(5-HT).svg *License*: unknown *Contributors*: User:NEUROtiker

GNU Free Documentation License Version 1.2, November 2002 Copyright (C) 2000,2001,2002 Free Software Foundation, Inc. 59 Temple Place, Suite 330, Boston, MA 02111-1307 USA Everyone is permitted to copy and distribute verbatim copies of this license document, but changing it is not allowed.

0. PREAMBLE

The purpose of this License is to make a manual, textbook, or other functional and useful document "free" in the sense of freedom: to assure everyone the effective freedom to copy and redistribute it, with or without modifying it, either commercially or noncommercially. Secondarily, this License preserves for the author and publisher a way to get credit for their work, while not being considered responsible for modifications made by others. This License is a kind of "copyleft", which means that derivative works of the document must themselves be free in the same sense. It complements the GNU General Public License, which is a copyleft license designed for free software. We have designed this License in order to use it for manuals for free software, because free software needs free documentation: a free program should come with manuals providing the same freedoms that the software does. But this License is not limited to software manuals; it can be used for any textual work, regardless of subject matter or whether it is published as a printed book. We recommend this License principally for works whose purpose is instruction or reference.

1. APPLICABILITY AND DEFINITIONS

This License applies to any manual or other work, in any medium, that contains a notice placed by the copyright holder saying it can be distributed under the terms of this License. Such a notice grants a world-wide, royalty-free license, unlimited in duration, to use that work under the conditions stated herein. The "Document", below, refers to any such manual or work. Any member of the public is a licensee, and is addressed as "you". You accept the license if you copy, modify or distribute the work in a way requiring permission under copyright law. A "Modified Version" of the Document means any work containing the Document or a portion of it, either copied verbatim, or with modifications and/or translated into another language. A "Secondary Section" is a named appendix or a front-matter section of the Document that deals exclusively with the relationship of the publishers or authors of the Document to the Document's overall subject (or to related matters) and contains nothing that could fall directly within that overall subject. (Thus, if the Document is in part a textbook of mathematics, a Secondary Section may not explain any mathematics.) The relationship could be a matter of historical connection with the subject or with related matters, or of legal, commercial, philosophical, ethical or political position regarding them. The "Invariant Sections" are certain Secondary Sections whose titles are designated, as being those of Invariant Sections, in the notice that says that the Document is released under this License. If a section does not fit the above definition of Secondary then it is not allowed to be designated as Invariant. The Document may contain zero Invariant Sections. If the Document does not identify any Invariant Sections then there are none. The "Cover Texts" are certain short passages of text that are listed, as Front-Cover Texts or Back-Cover Texts, in the notice that says that the Document is released under this License. A Front-Cover Text may be at most 5 words, and a Back-Cover Text may be at most 25 words. A "Transparent" copy of the Document means a machine-readable copy, represented in a format whose specification is available to the general public, that is suitable for revising the document straightforwardly with generic text editors or (for images composed of pixels) generic paint programs or (for drawings) some widely available drawing editor, and that is suitable for input to text formatters or for automatic translation to a variety of formats suitable for input to text formatters. A copy made in an otherwise Transparent file format whose markup, or absence of markup, has been arranged to thwart or discourage subsequent modification by readers is not Transparent. An image format is not Transparent if used for any substantial amount of text. A copy that is not "Transparent" is called "Opaque". Examples of suitable formats for Transparent copies include plain ASCII without markup, Texinfo input format, LaTeX input format, SGML or XML using a publicly available DTD, and standard-conforming simple HTML, PostScript or PDF designed for human modification. Examples of transparent image formats include PNG, XCF and JPG. Opaque formats include proprietary formats that can be read and edited only by proprietary word processors, SGML or XML for which the DTD and/or processing tools are not generally available, and the machine-generated HTML, PostScript or PDF produced by some word processors for output purposes only. The "Title Page" means, for a printed book, the title page itself, plus such following pages as are needed to hold, legibly, the material this License requires to appear in the title page. For works in formats which do not have any title page as such, "Title Page" means the text near the most prominent appearance of the work's title, preceding the beginning of the body of the text. A section "Entitled XYZ" means a named subunit of the Document whose title either is precisely XYZ or contains XYZ in parentheses following text that translates XYZ in another language. (Here XYZ stands for a specific section name mentioned below, such as "Acknowledgements", "Dedications", "Endorsements", or "History".) To "Preserve the Title" of such a section when you modify the Document means that it remains a section "Entitled XYZ" according to this definition. The Document may include Warranty Disclaimers next to the notice which states that this License applies to the Document. These Warranty Disclaimers are considered to be included by reference in this License, but only as regards disclaiming warranties: any other implication that these Warranty Disclaimers may have is void and has no effect on the meaning of this License.

2. VERBATIM COPYING

You may copy and distribute the Document in any medium, either commercially or noncommercially, provided that this License, the copyright notices, and the license notice saying this License applies to the Document are reproduced in all copies, and that you add no other conditions whatsoever to those of this License. You may not use technical measures to obstruct or control the reading or further copying of the copies you make or distribute. However, you may accept compensation in exchange for copies. If you distribute a large enough number of copies you must also follow the conditions in section 3. You may also lend copies, under the same conditions stated above, and you may publicly display copies.

3. COPYING IN QUANTITY

If you publish printed copies (or copies in media that commonly have printed covers) of the Document, numbering more than 100, and the Document's license notice requires Cover Texts, you must enclose the copies in covers that carry, clearly and legibly, all these Cover Texts: Front-Cover Texts on the front cover, and Back-Cover Texts on the back cover. Both covers must also clearly and legibly identify you as the publisher of these copies. The front cover must present the full title with all words of the title equally prominent and visible. You may add other material on the covers in addition. Copying with changes limited to the covers, as long as they preserve the title of the Document and satisfy these conditions, can be treated as verbatim copying in other respects. If the required texts for either cover are too voluminous to fit legibly, you should put the first ones listed (as many as fit reasonably) on the actual cover, and continue the rest onto adjacent pages. If you publish or distribute Opaque copies of the Document numbering more than 100, you must either include a machine-readable Transparent copy along with each Opaque copy, or state in or with each Opaque copy a computer-network location from which the general network-using public has access to download using public-standard network protocols a complete Transparent copy of the Document, free of added material. If you use the latter option, you must take reasonably prudent steps, when you begin distribution of Opaque copies in quantity, to ensure that this Transparent copy will remain thus accessible at the stated location until at least one year after the last time you distribute an Opaque copy (directly or through your agents or retailers) of that edition to the public. It is requested, but not required, that you contact the authors of the Document well before redistributing any large number of copies, to give them a chance to provide you with an updated version of the Document.

4. MODIFICATIONS

You may copy and distribute a Modified Version of the Document under the conditions of sections 2 and 3 above, provided that you release the Modified Version under precisely this License, with the Modified Version filling the role of the Document, thus licensing distribution and modification of the Modified Version to whoever possesses a copy of it. In addition, you must do these things in the Modified Version: A. Use in the Title Page (and on the covers, if any) a title distinct from that of the Document, and from those of previous versions (which should, if there were any, be listed in the History section of the Document). You may use the same title as a previous version if the original publisher of that version gives permission. B. List on the Title Page, as authors, one or more persons or entities responsible for authorship of the modifications in the Modified Version, together with at least five of the principal authors of the Document (all of its principal authors, if it has fewer than five), unless they release you from this requirement. C. State on the Title page the name of the publisher of the Modified Version, as the publisher. D. Preserve all the copyright notices of the Document. E. Add an appropriate copyright notice for your modifications adjacent to the other copyright notices. F. Include, immediately after the copyright notices, a license notice giving the public permission to use the Modified Version under the terms of this License, in the form shown in the Addendum below. G. Preserve in that license notice the full lists of Invariant Sections and required Cover Texts given in the Document's license notice. H. Include an unaltered copy of this License. I. Preserve the section Entitled "History", Preserve its Title, and add to it an item stating at least the title, year, new authors, and publisher of the Modified Version as given on the Title Page. If there is no section Entitled "History" in the Document, create one stating the title, year, authors, and publisher of the Document as given on its Title Page, then add an item describing the Modified Version as stated in the previous sentence. J. Preserve the network location, if any, given in the Document for public access to a Transparent copy of the Document, and likewise the network locations given in the Document for previous versions it was based on. These may be placed in the "History" section. You may omit a network location for a work that was published at least four years before the Document itself, or if the original publisher of the version it refers to gives permission. K. For any section Entitled "Acknowledgements" or "Dedications", Preserve the Title of the section, and preserve in the section all the substance and tone of each of the contributor acknowledgements and/or dedications given therein. L. Preserve all the Invariant Sections of the Document, unaltered in their text and in their titles. Section numbers or the equivalent are not considered part of the section titles. M. Delete any section Entitled "Endorsements". Such a section may not be included in the Modified Version. N. Do not retitle any existing section to be Entitled "Endorsements" or to conflict in title with any Invariant Section. O. Preserve any Warranty Disclaimers. If the Modified Version includes new front-matter sections or appendices that qualify as Secondary Sections and contain no material copied from the Document, you may at your option designate some or all of these sections as invariant. To do this, add their titles to the list of Invariant Sections in the Modified Version's license notice. These titles must be distinct from any other section titles. You may add a section Entitled "Endorsements", provided it contains nothing but endorsements of your Modified Version by various parties--for example, statements of peer review or that the text has been approved by an organization as the authoritative definition of a standard. You may add a passage of up to five words as a Front-Cover Text, and a passage of up to 25 words as a Back-Cover Text, to the end of the list of Cover Texts in the Modified Version. Only one passage of Front-Cover Text and one of Back-Cover Text may be added by (or through arrangements made by) any one entity. If the Document already includes a cover text for the same cover, previously added by you or by arrangement made by the same entity you are acting on behalf of, you may not add another; but you may replace the old one, on explicit permission from the previous publisher that added the old one. The author(s) and publisher(s) of the Document do not by this License give permission to use their names for publicity for or to assert or imply endorsement of any Modified Version.

5. COMBINING DOCUMENTS

You may combine the Document with other documents released under this License, under the terms defined in section 4 above for modified versions, provided that you include in the combination all of the Invariant Sections of all of the original documents, unmodified, and list them all as Invariant Sections of your combined work in its license notice, and that you preserve all their Warranty Disclaimers. The combined work need only contain one copy of this License, and multiple identical Invariant Sections may be replaced with a single copy. If there are multiple Invariant Sections with the same name but different contents, make the title of each such section unique by adding at the end of it, in parentheses, the name of the original author or publisher of that section if known, or else a unique number. Make the same adjustment to the section titles in the list of Invariant Sections in the license notice of the combined work. In the combination, you must combine any sections Entitled "History" in the various original documents, forming one section Entitled "History"; likewise combine any sections Entitled "Acknowledgements", and any sections Entitled "Dedications". You must delete all sections Entitled "Endorsements".

6. COLLECTIONS OF DOCUMENTS

You may make a collection consisting of the Document and other documents released under this License, and replace the individual copies of this License in the various documents with a single copy that is included in the collection, provided that you follow the rules of this License for verbatim copying of each of the documents in all other respects. You may extract a single document from such a collection, and distribute it individually under this License, provided you insert a copy of this License into the extracted document, and follow this License in all other respects regarding verbatim copying of that document.

7. AGGREGATION WITH INDEPENDENT WORKS

A compilation of the Document or its derivatives with other separate and independent documents or works, in or on a volume of a storage or distribution medium, is called an "aggregate" if the copyright resulting from the compilation is not used to limit the legal rights of the compilation's users beyond what the individual works permit. When the Document is included in an aggregate, this License does not apply to the other works in the aggregate which are not themselves derivative works of the Document. If the Cover Text requirement of section 3 is applicable to these copies of the Document, then if the Document is less than one half of the entire aggregate, the Document's Cover Texts may be placed on covers that bracket the Document within the aggregate, or the electronic equivalent of covers if the Document is in electronic form. Otherwise they must appear on printed covers that bracket the whole aggregate.

8. TRANSLATION

Translation is considered a kind of modification, so you may distribute translations of the Document under the terms of section 4. Replacing Invariant Sections with translations requires special permission from their copyright holders, but you may include translations of some or all Invariant Sections in addition to the original versions of these Invariant Sections. You may include a translation of this License, and all the license notices in the Document, and any Warranty Disclaimers, provided that you also include the original English version of this License and the original versions of those notices and disclaimers. In case of a disagreement between the translation and the original version of this License or a notice or disclaimer, the original version will prevail. If a section in the Document is Entitled "Acknowledgements", "Dedications", or "History", the requirement (section 4) to Preserve its Title (section 1) will typically require changing the actual title.

9. TERMINATION

You may not copy, modify, sublicense, or distribute the Document except as expressly provided for under this License. Any other attempt to copy, modify, sublicense or distribute the Document is void, and will automatically terminate your rights under this License. However, parties who have received copies, or rights, from you under this License will not have their licenses terminated so long as such parties remain in full compliance.

10. FUTURE REVISIONS OF THIS LICENSE

The Free Software Foundation may publish new, revised versions of the GNU Free Documentation License from time to time. Such new versions will be similar in spirit to the present version, but may differ in detail to address new problems or concerns. See http://www.gnu.org/copyleft/. Each version of the License is given a distinguishing version number. If the Document specifies that a particular numbered version of this License "or any later version" applies to it, you have the option of following the terms and conditions either of that specified version or of any later version that has been published (not as a draft) by the Free Software Foundation. If the Document does not specify a version number of this License, you may choose any version ever published (not as a draft) by the Free Software Foundation. ADDENDUM: How to use this License for your documents To use this License in a document you have written, include a copy of the License in the document and put the following copyright and license notices just after the title page: Copyright (c) YEAR YOUR NAME. Permission is granted to copy, distribute and/or modify this document under the terms of the GNU Free Documentation License, Version 1.2 or any later version published by the Free Software Foundation; with no Invariant Sections, no Front-Cover Texts, and no Back-Cover Texts. A copy of the license is included in the section entitled "GNU Free Documentation License". If you have Invariant Sections, Front-Cover Texts and Back-Cover Texts, replace the "with...Texts." line with this: with the Invariant Sections being LIST THEIR TITLES, with the Front-Cover Texts being LIST, and with the Back-Cover Texts being LIST. If you have Invariant Sections without Cover Texts, or some other combination of the three, merge those two alternatives to suit the situation. If your document contains nontrivial examples of program code, we recommend releasing these examples in parallel under your choice of free software license, such as the GNU General Public License, to permit their use in free software.

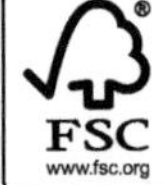

MIX
Papier aus verantwortungsvollen Quellen
Paper from responsible sources
FSC® C105338

Printed by Books on Demand GmbH, Norderstedt / Germany

Segmentation Contractions

Please note that the content of this book primarily consists of articles available from Wikipedia or other free sources online. Segmentation contractions (or movements) are a type of gastric motility. Unlike peristalsis, which predominates in the esophagus, segmentation contractions occur in the large intestine and small intestine, while predominating in the latter. While peristalsis involves one-way motion in the caudal direction, segmentation contractions move chyme in both directions, which allows greater mixing with the secretions of the intestines.

978-613-7-88792-9

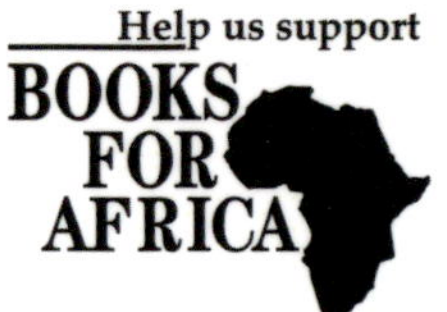

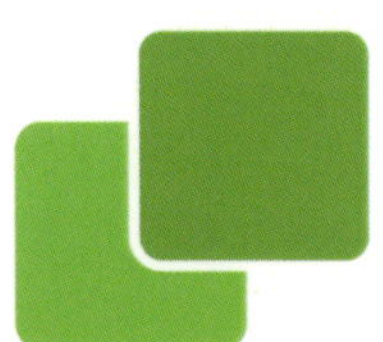